Janene Carey is a freelance writer, editor and academic. Previously, she was employed as a journalist, sub-editor and acting editor with her local newspaper, *The Armidale Express*. She has a PhD in writing, and her work has been published in national newspapers, magazines and literary journals, including *The Sydney Morning Herald*, *The Sun-Herald*, OUTBACK *magazine*, *Australian Book Review*, TEXT and *Perilous Adventures*. Her website is www.janenecarey.com

A HOSPITAL BED AT HOME

FAMILY STORIES OF CAREGIVING FROM
DIAGNOSIS TO DEATH

JANENE CAREY

TABLELANDS PRESS

ARMIDALE, NSW

Tablelands Press
5 Highlands Rd Dumaresq NSW 2350

National Library of Australia Cataloguing-in-Publication data:
Carey, Janene Patricia
A hospital bed at home : family stories of caregiving from diagnosis to death /
Janene Carey.
ISBN 9780992423605 (paperback)
ISBN 9780992423612 (ebook : Kindle)
ISBN 9780992423629 (ebook : epub)
Terminal care–Australia–Anecdotes.
Caregivers–Australia–Anecdotes.
Terminally ill–Australia–Death.
Palliative treatment–Australia.
Dewey Number: 362.1750994

Cover design: Trish Donald
Cover photo: theoccasionalgardener.com

This book was produced using PressBooks.com with PDF rendering by Prince
XML. Typefaces are Cinzel and Sorts Mill Goudy.

Author website: www.janenecarey.com

This book is lovingly dedicated to my mother, Pat Carey, a warm-hearted, creative and skilful woman, always active, always giving.
11 November 1940 – 14 November 2006

CONTENTS

INTRODUCTION

In the nine years spanning my mother's initial diagnosis of breast cancer and her death in November 2006, people often told me how much they admired her 'fighting spirit' – her determination to conquer the disease that kept returning to ravage her. I didn't like the martial imagery but found myself employing it too, just in a different way. From where I was standing, the cancer was the fighter, a relentless opponent, always coming at her with another jabbing punch. To her breast, chest, hip, groin, then the knock-out blow, to her brain.

Mum's chief defence was an unflagging but anxiety-ridden optimism; her attitude was quite literally never-say-die. As the number of tumour battle sites mounted, I could see that the odds were stacked against her, but she never reasoned in terms of probabilities. She took refuge in the good news stories told by survivors, she quested after the miracle cure that would confound medical science, she prayed to God for healing. Was this courage, I wondered? This refusal to accept the most likely outcome, this frenetic hunt for an escape clause?

As her condition worsened, maintaining the fiction of a happy ending became more difficult. By March 2006, she was troubled by a growing list of distressing symptoms that her medical advisors did not seem to be able to fix. She fretted about whether she should see another doctor, someone 'less negative' than her oncologist, who had told her quite bluntly that she would not get better. I refrained from mentioning that not only did the oncologist think she would 'not get better', he had informed me that she would 'get progressively worse' and only had a few months to live. During these kinds of conversations with my mother, I would feel like I was groping in the dark, trying to gauge her willingness to talk openly, wishing I had a more finely honed instinct for knowing what to say and what to leave unsaid.

As it happened, Mum lived for five months longer than her oncologist had predicted. However, during this time she was in a state of piteous dependence: bedridden, unable to walk, talk properly or feed herself. For the last three months she was in a nursing home, wasting away to a husk. Even so, when the doctor told her in November that she had contracted pneumonia and he planned to let it run its course, she was not at all inclined to see it as a merciful release. Her body tensed with fear and her face spoke her anguish.

The registered nurse on duty that day was Deb, a whippet-thin blonde whose brisk efficient manner hid a core of genuine kindness. She took me aside and said that the strength of my mother's reaction had taken both her and the doctor by surprise. 'She was so upset. She was horrified. It made me realise that we'll have to change how we're interacting with her.'

'What do you mean?'

'Well, most people who move into a nursing home understand that they're going to die here. They often make jokes about it, and so do the staff.'

'You mean you'll have to stop saying, "So you're still here, then?" when you walk into her room in the morning?' I asked.

'Yes,' said Deb, laughing. 'That's exactly what I mean.'

I rang my brother Michael, marvelling that Mum was still rejecting the idea of dying even as her body was shutting down its last remaining functions. 'I don't think she's ever going to accept it,' I said.

'Well, I wouldn't either.'

His comment made me wonder why I was still clinging to the expectation that my mother should meet this coming death with serenity. She'd never been serene. She would die as she had lived.

Caring for someone who is terminally ill is not a subject that is easily broached in Australian society, and so, like most people, I was unprepared for the overwhelming physical, emotional and psychological challenges it entails. I had assumed that I would somehow rise to the occasion but instead found that I was sinking under the stresses, ground down by worry, injury, lack of sleep and anticipatory grief. Writing about what I was going through, often in the middle of the night, was part of how I coped.

When it was over, I felt impelled to investigate other people's experiences. I decided that I would write a book of stories about what it is like to be a caregiver during the weeks, months and years that can stretch between the day someone you love is diagnosed with an incurable, fatal disease and the day of his or her death. It was immensely reassuring for me to find that other carers struggled, as I did, to do the job well, and to realise that we had faced many of the same difficulties. Tracing the trajectory of each story biographically helped me to recognise that carers and patients bring to their roles the full gamut of typically human strengths and weaknesses, plus all the complications of their pre-existing relationship. To find the situation extremely difficult at times is entirely normal; to respond imperfectly at times is entirely understandable. I felt a great load of residual guilt lift from my shoulders as I wrote.

The stories in *A Hospital Bed at Home* show how particular individuals have dealt with the awesome responsibility of overseeing the journey toward death of someone they love. I hope that these true stories will help caregivers – past, present and future – understand that other people have trodden a similar path, found it just as tangled and circuitous, yet managed to forge a way through that worked for themselves and their families. I hope the stories also serve to increase understanding and empathy in the general community, and among health professionals and policy-makers, about the problems faced by family carers and the kinds of support they may need.

Janene Carey

KATHERINE

In Australia, fewer than one in three expected deaths takes place outside an institution, but eighty per cent of people say they would rather die at home.

Home Hospice

I firmly believe that most people, given the opportunity, would prefer to die in familiar surroundings, amongst treasured possessions, cared for by people they know and love. The fact that it occurs so rarely is, I believe, less to do with the dying, and more to do with the living. The physical and mental strength required to nurse and oversee the deterioration and death of a loved one is incredible.

Katherine Baden's brother, Don

When Hugh Baden realised he was terminally ill, he took steps to ensure that the months ahead would unfold in accordance with his wishes. He informed his wife Katherine that he wanted no one to come to the house, apart from family. He visited his solicitor and drew up an Advance Care Directive, stipulating the kind of treatment he would accept in various circumstances and clearly stating his intention to be cared for at home until he died.

Flipping through this document during my second interview with Katherine, eighteen months after she had successfully completed a task that pushed her to her absolute physical and emotional limit, I found myself wondering what my mother would have made of it. Faced with these confronting irreversible conditions, would she have chosen life regardless, and ticked yes for the most active of medical interventions to prolong her existence? What if, from the vantage point of full command of her faculties, she could have seen into her future and understood that it was her fate to become permanently mildly demented, unable to remember things or reason clearly; permanently unable to speak meaningfully; totally cared for by others; bedridden, unable to wash, feed, or dress herself?

Would she still have wanted to live? Would she still have expected us to care for her at home?

Hugh Baden's Advance Care Directive indicated that he wanted no life-sustaining treatments. In a handwritten comment, he noted that he might have chosen differently if he hadn't known that he would still be facing the lung cancer afterwards.

'I wonder what my mum would have put,' I say to Katherine. 'If she'd been given something like this to fill out.'

I pause, realising just how unlikely it was that Mum would ever have wished to contemplate the possibilities listed on the form.

'I think she would have felt that any bit of life was better than none,' I say.

But of course I can't be sure, because we never discussed it.

RETREAT TO THE
CASTLE

A few kilometres from the town of Armidale in northern
New South Wales, a gravel driveway sidles around the
curve of a small hill and ends in a yard of barking dogs at
the back of a low dark-brick home. Hugh and Katherine
Baden came to live on this property, one hundred and
sixty acres of undulating grazing land, in 1968. Throughout the decades that followed they wove themselves into
the fabric of the community: working, volunteering,
socialising, pursuing various hobbies, putting three children through the local schools.

In November 2005, five months before he died, Hugh
Baden announced that he didn't want any more visitors.
'Only family,' he said. 'Nobody else.' Katherine had to tell
friends of twenty, thirty, forty years' standing not to come

to the house. Many people found it hard to understand. They thought they should be an exception to the rule: they rang up and asked to come just for ten minutes, to bring a meal, to give Hugh a hug, to sit with him, to say goodbye.

'Don't even come up the driveway,' Katherine told them. 'It sets the dogs off and Hugh gets angry and there's enough stress in the house already.'

Hugh was well liked, particularly by those who appreciate incisive intelligence coupled with sardonic humour. An agricultural scientist whose career had ridden, if not exactly on the sheep's back, certainly on the parasites they carry internally, he was regarded as a maverick: someone who had built a formidable reputation as a researcher despite refusing to do a PhD.

'He started out helping with experiments and went right up to senior principal research scientist,' Katherine informs me, her voice warm with pride and respect. 'I think he was a bit of a larrikin – he'd yahoo around the paddocks with the blokes, have motorbike races up and down the railway lines. Someone said to me once, "Hugh never seems to do any work!" But he was one of these people who didn't need much sleep. He'd spend four or five hours on his papers at night then he'd come to bed, wake me up, and tell me what he'd been doing.'

I laugh incredulously – I would murder anyone who

made a habit of waking me at two a.m. for a chat – but Katherine gives no indication of harbouring a grudge. She just adds that she always found it easy to fall asleep but Hugh needed to unwind before he could manage it.

Although small talk, like doctoral study, was another thing Hugh didn't bother with, a facility with words and a gift for spicing yarns and discussion of current events with peppercorns of dry wit meant that he could be great company. Katherine says when he set out to be amusing, Hugh could have people falling off their chairs with laughter. She thinks his talent as a raconteur blinded friends and colleagues to the fact that he had to make an effort to engage socially. He was essentially an introvert. Interacting with people drained him and he needed time alone to recharge.

When Hugh got sick, this tendency to find people exhausting became more pronounced. They gave him unwanted advice, asked too many questions, stayed too long. His home was his refuge, his castle. The ban on visitors was his way of pulling up the drawbridge. Henceforth his trusted companion, Katherine, was to be the keeper of the gate and handmaiden to his needs.

The details of Katherine's story about looking after Hugh unfold gradually, in a series of conversations. A mutual friend brokers our first contact. We have moved in overlapping social circles for years without encountering each other. We have a long talk on the phone; afterwards

I write up pages of notes punctuated by question marks. Our first meeting takes place at her home a few weeks later. Katherine greets me at the door, a tall, vigorous-looking woman in her sixties with a strong, frank face. We walk through her immaculate house to the family room and settle ourselves on the plush leather sofas. I get the impression that normally she is brisk and decisive about things but that today she is feeling uncharacteristically irresolute, unsure whether she's made the right decision in agreeing to talk to me. She tells me that yesterday she rang her brother and said, 'I'm in meltdown. I don't think I can do this.' Her anxiety is so obvious that I leave my voice recorder in my bag for the whole of our first interview, figuring that plonking it on the table between us would be a brutal conversation stopper.

She married Hugh when she was twenty-two years old. At the time, she was working as a primary school teacher. She was also the official Mayoress of Benalla; it was her job to accompany her widowed mother, the Mayor, to public functions. Hugh started out as a teacher, too, of high school science, but found it boring, so as soon as he'd done the three years required of Commonwealth scholarship holders he applied for a job at CSIRO and the couple moved to Armidale.

Katherine continued working as a teacher, on and off, until 1997. Hugh applied for voluntary redundancy from CSIRO in 1996 when it looked like his section was going to close down. Katherine's retirement activities included learning mah-jong, going to the gym, playing bridge and joining groups dedicated to sewing, bushwalking, talking about books and considering spiritual matters. Hugh took up one new activity – competitive shooting – but didn't so much retire as become self-employed: marking theses, editing scientific papers, and acting as a scientific adviser for a company that made products for controlling worms in sheep and cattle. As a consultant, Hugh was able to retain the aspects of his previous job that he had most enjoyed – working with farmers, being at the cutting edge of research, attending international conferences – and jettison the parts he had most disliked: bureaucracy, organisational politics and the Monday-to-Friday routine.

One morning in July 2004, Hugh woke to find a lump the size of a golf ball protruding from the side of his face. Although the parotid tumour was never conclusively linked to the lung cancer that was diagnosed a year later, the treatment regime of surgical excision followed by five weeks of radiotherapy in Sydney marked the beginning of a rollercoaster ride of fear, hope and worry for the Baden family.

For six months it seemed everything was going to be fine; the worst was behind them. Then Hugh went back to his GP to report that each day, at around three p.m., he would run a high temperature and sweat profusely. After months of investigating possibilities like Ross River virus and Chronic Fatigue Syndrome, and ordering tests and x-rays that revealed nothing, the doctor phoned on the 27th of July 2005 and asked Hugh to come and see him that afternoon to discuss the results of a recent chest scan. He added that Hugh should bring his wife.

Hugh was sixty-three years old and had been a smoker for forty years, but the news that he had lung cancer still took them by surprise.

'We just sat there. I couldn't believe it. Because there'd always been this family joke that Hugh would die of lung cancer. We always joked about the most appalling things. We said he'd die of cancer but it never really occurred to us that he actually would. His mother was a chain-smoker and she lived into her seventies and died of a heart attack. We all thought, well, Hugh's made of the same stuff.'

The Sydney-based oncologist who visited Armidale regularly told Hugh that his cancer was incurable, but said chemotherapy would slow the progression of the disease. Hugh had two rounds of chemotherapy and the tumours shrank by fifty per cent, prompting the doctor to announce that if the trend continued, Hugh might go into full remission. However, a month later the tumours had regrown to larger than their original size.

Hugh and Katherine went to Brisbane for a second opinion about treatment options. The specialist was amazed that Hugh had been able to walk from a nearby motel to the hospital. He showed them x-rays of the large tumours in both lungs and explained that they were inoperable because they were too close to the spine.

'We should have been depressed,' comments Katherine. 'But we found it reassuring. It was the same diagnosis that we had been given by the Sydney specialist.'

The Badens' acceptance of Hugh's condition as terminal was something else that other people found hard to understand. It wasn't the 'right' attitude. The prevailing cultural norm is to regard those with cancer as soldiers fighting a war, brandishing the indispensable weapons of hope and positive thinking. People seemed to think it was their duty to act as recruiting sergeants and push Hugh forward to the front line, equipped with whatever was available in the alternative medicine armoury.

Katherine describes her amazement at the liberties people took in dispensing advice: 'We went to a birthday dinner, and individuals kept taking Hugh aside and telling him that they knew how he could be cured. Someone mentioned a chap who waved his hands above you and miraculously healed you of anything at all. Then there were the folk who gave us books on beating cancer. Everybody wanted to tell us what to do. It was incredible how insistent and repetitive the advice was! They told Hugh over and over again, as if he was a slow learner and he hadn't understood it the first time.'

It occurs to me that someone like Hugh, a scientist who had spent years dealing with reality in a logical and rational manner, would find it hard to tolerate exhortations to believe in miracle cures and to adopt courses of action based on magical thinking. I ask Katherine whether other people's insistence that a cure was possible had ever provoked Hugh to argue the point, but she said no. 'He'd just let them blather on, but he'd come home and he'd be hugely angry. It really was harassment,' says Katherine. 'We felt emotionally violated. The fact that it was done with the best of intentions was no consolation.'

Another piece of proffered advice concerned how to spend the remaining time. 'Why don't you travel, or go to the coast?' a woman said to Katherine. 'You've got this short time frame of maybe three months before he gets sick again. Do something!'

Katherine went home and told her husband about this suggestion. 'What would you like to do?' she asked him.

He responded with derision. 'I've travelled overseas three times a year for most of my working life. I've seen fifty-two countries. And I hate going to the coast. You've always known that. The thing I like best is being at home. So please, can I have the privilege of being happy at home?'

'Fine!' shrugged Katherine. Although she had been left behind for most of those work trips when the children were small, there had been a sabbatical year in Maine and a research program in Fiji that the family had enjoyed together; and during the last ten years she and Hugh had been camping in the Kimberley region of Western Australia, caught the Tran-Siberian Express across Russia, Mongolia and China with a group of friends from the bushwalking club, and cruised the Inside Passage of Alaska. She could understand why Hugh didn't see any need to cram more travel experiences into the time he had left.

As soon as Hugh knew that his condition was terminal, he arranged to see a lawyer, to make a clear statement of his intention to be cared for at home, and to die there. This didn't imply an acceptance of death as imminent.

'We saw this as being like writing a will. Important, but something to be used in the future. The far distant future, we hoped,' Katherine explains.

I ask Katherine how she had felt about taking on this responsibility. Did she know what she was letting herself in for? She replies that she gave her consent freely and went into it with her eyes open. However, she doubts whether Hugh would have cared for her in the same way, if their positions had been reversed.

'No, I don't think he would have done it for me. I think he might have been too impatient to cope with it all.'

She muses about whether female social conditioning might explain why she accepted Hugh's request so readily, and then remembers something.

'When I was twelve, my father died of bowel cancer and my mother looked after him at home. It wasn't so common in those days. Seeing her cope with it – I guess that's why I felt that I could do it for Hugh.'

A child's view of what was involved in caring for a sick husband may not have been the most reliable template for what lay ahead of her. Katherine had assumed that it would be just a variation on the maternal role, but in fact she found herself caught up in the most stressful experience of her life.

'I had assumed that I could manage on my own. I really did think that looking after someone like that would be like looking after a baby. You would be sleep deprived and feed them and pat them on the back and sure, it's emotionally demanding, but you can cope. But it's really not like that at all. I was pushed to my absolute limit, physically and emotionally. And that's why I ended up with all these people coming to help me, and my brother living in the house for two months. I couldn't have managed, otherwise.'

The palliative care nurse started visiting early on, while Hugh still felt well enough to manage his regular activities. 'We both thought it was a bit premature, even though we'd seen the lawyer. She wanted details about our family, where they lived, what our medical cover was. We filled in forms saying how often we wanted her to come and what her role would be. It was confronting, but we had to face the reality of what lay ahead.'

It is a common misconception that palliative care is

synonymous with end-of-life care. Ideally, palliative care begins soon after the diagnosis of an incurable, life-threatening disease and goes beyond the relief of physical suffering to include the psychological, emotional, social and spiritual well-being of the entire family. According to the World Health Organisation, palliative care should support patients to live as actively as possible and help the family cope both during the illness and after their loved one has died.

Katherine believes the palliative care services that she received in Armidale were marvellous. She tells me about going to a bereavement support group and feeling impatient with the moanings of another widow who, mistrusting the care available locally, had carted her husband off to Sydney, only to find that in the big city he was treated as just another number. Katherine had roundly informed this woman that the services in Armidale couldn't be better, and cited her own, radically different, experience. Doctors and nurses made weekly home visits. Respite care was organised for her. When she went to the doctor's surgery to get a prescription, the usual fee was waived. 'We don't charge the Badens,' was the message relayed in a whisper to the person on the desk.

While she could still leave Hugh for periods, Katherine coped as the sole carer, though it made her anxious. 'I was worried that he would fall over while I was away. We would discuss whether he could manage without walking about. I went to the gym at eight a.m. for an hour. I often walked for an hour at night. I still played competition bridge three times a week. I needed to go out, but I was racked with guilt. Would he fall? Would he go out to the paddocks? Would he commit suicide? Two of his uncles did that when they had cancer.' She describes this as a period of doubt and unexpressed anger. 'It was difficult for me, not knowing what to do. It was tiring and I felt alone.'

Broken sleep was a problem for both of them. Hugh woke up frequently during the night, wanting help to turn over, to get a drink, to go to the toilet. Even when he slept, the bedroom was not peaceful. He talked loudly; he was plagued by nightmares. Katherine would snap to alertness to check if he was okay. Hugh's eyes became a problem: he couldn't read any more and his distance vision became blurred. Katherine got a stack of glasses from Vinnies for him to try. They found a pair that improved things but his vision changed again and the problem returned.

Despite the broken nights and the difficulties with vision and balance, Katherine thought Hugh was doing remarkably well. It was a trip to Brisbane to visit a new grandchild that made her realise just how ill he had become.

'The flight was a disaster. It debilitated him. He went to our daughter's home and just lay on a mattress on the floor. His eyes were flat and dull and he just lay there motionless. Kerryn was frantic. She said, "Dad is dying! Look at him!" She wanted me to do something, to call a doctor. I refused. I suggested we leave him in peace. He spent most of the weekend like that, prostrate.'

On the last night of the visit, Hugh roused himself to have an evening meal at the home of his eldest son, Alan. Both sons and their wives were there. Hugh ate very little, and after the first course commented that he wanted to say something. The tension was palpable. He told them he expected to die before Christmas and said that he wanted to give each of them $200,000.

Alan and his brother Paul refused the money outright. Katherine and Hugh left. They returned to their daughter's house, where Hugh's offer was again vehemently rejected.

The family had understood the severity of Hugh's illness, but this pronouncement of his impending death was shocking. 'He basically said: "I'm going to die, I'll give you some money, and now we're going home." The kids were appalled. We had the most horrendous fight over this. They couldn't believe that he'd been in Brisbane for three days and just before he left he made these dramatic and emotionally charged statements and then went off without giving them any time to react and adjust. It took me about five phone calls to each of them for everyone to agree that it had all been mishandled. They wanted their father alive. They didn't want the news of his death and the offer of money, together, as if somehow the money compensated for the death.'

Back in Armidale, the palliative care nurse suggested putting a hospital bed in the family room off the kitchen. Hugh used this during the day, but slept with Katherine in their bedroom at night. Eventually he couldn't walk down the hall. More equipment was provided: a light wheelchair to make the journey between the beds; a commode chair, to bring toileting facilities closer.

Katherine sent out Christmas cards containing the message that Hugh was seriously ill with advanced lung cancer. Communication between Hugh and his younger brothers, Stephen and Richard, had been sporadic as adults, so this was news to them. Each rang Katherine as soon as the letter arrived, asking to come for a weekend visit.

When Stephen came, Katherine made a point of absenting herself. 'I thought it was better to just leave them, so they could engage in whatever way they wanted to,' she explains. On her return she found Hugh lying with his eyes shut and his brother sitting quietly on the sofa nearby. She asked Stephen what had been happening while she was out. "Oh, I've been reading poetry to Hugh," he answered. Katherine would never have thought of doing such a thing herself, but she was absolutely delighted that Stephen, who has a beautiful speaking voice, had remembered Hugh's love of poetry.

Despite the years of infrequent contact, each brother's visit was both distinctive and successful. Richard, the youngest one, did a lot of work outside. Through the floor to ceiling windows that looked out over the back paddocks, Hugh could see his brother taking care of the chores and befriending the dogs. Richard came inside periodically and reported on his activities to Hugh, who would say "Yes!" in a relieved tone of voice and go back to sleep happily.

Stephen and Richard both returned after the initial weekend to spend a full week at Hugh and Katherine's house. Katherine says she cried when they left, 'Because I thought, they've connected to Hugh in their own individual way, in a way that I couldn't. They made this huge contribution to his peace of mind.'

From January onwards, Hugh's imminent demise was regularly predicted by the doctors. 'He would look as if he was dying but somehow he would rally. They said to me afterwards that it was being at home that kept him going. They said if you'd put him in hospital he would have died months ago. But real life going on around him all the time kept him stimulated.'

Katherine was beginning to feel ground down by the exhausting days and nights. 'Hugh would ask to go to bed at about seven-thirty. He didn't like being alone at this stage and he had a bell that he rang to get my attention. If I left him alone at night, even for five minutes, the bell would ring and he'd be asking when I was coming to bed. Mostly I was happy to sleep, even at seven-thirty. The days were so busy, physically and emotionally demanding, and we were awake a lot during the night.'

'The bed linen needed changing every day on both beds. It didn't matter what I did, bodily matter and fluid spread everywhere. We tried all kinds of sheeting, nappy-like underwear, anything that was suggested by chemists, nurses or doctors, but it was all in vain. I wondered how ghastly it must have been for him, how humiliating. This was one topic we never talked about. We went through the procedure in silence every day. I bathed him, changed his pyjamas and changed the bed sheets. His dignity carried him through. It was just something that had to be endured, as often as was needed.'

Word got out somehow about the heavy load that Katherine was carrying. Even now, she isn't sure how the respite services were organised. Someone must have seen that she needed help, and eventually it arrived in the unlikely guise of twelve strapping blokes on a rota system.

A female manager with Community Health rang from Sydney, insisting that Katherine persuade Hugh to accept care from other people. 'Tell him this help is for you, not him.' The woman pointed out that it wasn't a question of charity, as by looking after Hugh at home, Katherine was saving the health care system about $600 a day.

Hugh capitulated. However, the first respite care experience was almost the last. Hugh disliked having a strange woman sitting with him. He presumed that she would be like other women he had known, wanting to plague him with questions. How was he feeling? Was he comfortable? What was he thinking about?

In fact, says Katherine, this particular woman didn't say much at all. But Hugh announced he didn't want anyone except his wife looking after him. Katherine rang to cancel the respite care arrangement. Showing great perception, the local organiser asked whether Hugh would prefer men to come out and sit with him. This was the perfect solution. Hugh had worked in a male-dominated environment all his life and was most comfortable with its bluff good humour, emotional distance, and taciturn style of interaction. There were twelve different men who took it in turns to sit companionably but silently by Hugh's bedside, allowing Katherine to go to the gym and to play bridge several afternoons a week. Katherine refers to these men fondly as 'the blokes' and says every one of them was 'nothing less than excellent'.

She does report one little hiccup. The help being provided was actually supposed to be 'home help'. Katherine always had her house perfectly ordered before the blokes arrived, and one of them must have complained that there was no work to do. When asked to give them tasks to complete in her absence, she explained that she only wanted them to sit quietly. She didn't want them pottering around doing little jobs, even if Hugh was asleep. She wanted them to be visible, a presence in the room, in case he woke up. After this misunderstanding was resolved, the arrangement proceeded smoothly.

Other help was provided by family members. Their adult children took turns to visit on the weekends, flying down to Armidale on Saturday and leaving on Sunday at lunchtime. In the early days, the eldest grandchildren came too. 'They would play around the bed, climb up beside him, give him a hug. It was astonishing how easily they accepted Hugh's changed way of life.'

It was during a weekend visit by her daughter, Kerryn, on the 24th of January, when Katherine first wondered if she would be able to continue looking after Hugh on her own at night. Her sleep between the hours of midnight and three a.m. was regularly interrupted by his wild hallucinations. On this particular Saturday, Hugh got out of bed and fell down in the dressing room; when Katherine went to pick him up he bellowed that he was drowning in chocolate. His body was a complete dead weight, he was convinced that he was trapped in a river of sticky chocolate. Unable to lift him, Katherine called out for Kerryn, who was sleeping in the next room. Like Katherine, Kerryn is tall and fit, but it took their combined strength to get Hugh to his feet. Katherine suddenly realised that she'd got to the stage where she felt physically and psychologically unable to handle such crises by herself.

Kerryn made a list of all the hallucinations that Hugh suffered that night. He was firing gunshots down the hallway at an imaginary enemy. He was trying to get a drink of water from a mobile phone. He didn't know he was Hugh: he thought Hugh had disappeared and Katherine should get in touch with him. At one stage he didn't know who Katherine was, but he wanted whoever it was in the bed next to him to tell Katherine that she was a really good bloke. It was as if he was acting out his dreams, at full volume and with all the movements.

This kind of thing happened almost every night. Each hallucinatory dream would last about fifteen to twenty minutes, with Katherine struggling to wake Hugh up and bring him back to reality. 'If I kept at it long enough, or if I could get him to laugh, he'd suddenly snap out of it and say, "It's my mind, isn't it?" and I'd say, "Yes, it's your mind playing funny tricks".' They would then go back to sleep for about twenty minutes before the next episode began.

On Sunday, as Kerryn was leaving, she said, 'You know, Mum, I'm at home with three kids under five. I am flat out and sleep deprived. But I'm in paradise compared to you!'

Respite care allowed Katherine to maintain regular contact with groups of friends at social activities. She realised how concerned people were about her welfare when a casual remark she made at the bridge club brought play at her table to a complete standstill. In response to a comment from somebody about being hungry, Katherine had said, 'Oh! Well, I have this tremendous craving ... ' There was an immediate, attentive silence, then the solicitous query: 'What do you crave, Katherine?' Unfortunately, the object of Katherine's craving was not something her friends could give her. 'I crave sleep,' she announced. 'My every waking thought is taken up with – when will I next sleep?'

She tells me that on one occasion she lay down on her bed when a respite carer came to sit with Hugh, and she went to sleep for half an hour. However, she decided not to make a habit of it. 'I woke up and I thought: this is ridiculous. I've got things I've got to do and if I sleep in the daytime I can't get those things done and everything's going to fall apart. You have to answer phone calls and things have to be bought and washing has to be brought in. So you really have to be disciplined to keep it all going. To keep the house tidy and immaculate, because that's how you like to live.'

Hugh would doze lightly during the day, free of the terrors that assailed him at night. As his bed was in the centre of the house, he was able to drift in and out of conversations, sometimes quite disconcertingly. Katherine remembers a particular occasion when Hugh seemed completely oblivious to the discussion she was having with her youngest son, Paul, and his wife. She said, 'I've got this fantastic quote, this is what life is all about.' She read it out and invited them to tell her what they thought. Hugh opened his eyes and said, 'It's absolute rubbish.' Katherine was understandably offended. Hugh explained that he agreed with the sentiment of the quote; it was the wording – a corruption of verses from the Bible – to which he objected. The passage, from Ecclesiastes 9:11-12, was later read at Hugh's funeral service in its original, untainted form:

> I returned, and saw under the sun, that the race is not to the swift, nor the battle to the strong, neither yet bread to the wise, nor yet riches to men of understanding, nor yet favour to men of skill: but time and chance happeneth to them all. For man also knoweth not his time: as the fishes that are taken in an evil net, and as the birds that are caught in the snare; so are the sons of men snared in an evil time, when it falleth suddenly upon them.

Towards the end of February, Katherine's older brother, Don, a retired veterinarian living in Melbourne, decided it was time to override his sister's protestations that she was managing and didn't need his help. He rang and told her that he had booked flights to come and stay and would be arriving in three days.

'I left home knowing I'd be away for six to eight weeks, possibly longer – I planned to stay until Hugh died. I knew Katherine was struggling and it would be good for her to have someone to share the load. I thought Hugh would accept me, if only because the alternative was hospitalisation,' Don explained to me in a letter.

Katherine was happy to be persuaded. 'I had such a close relationship with him when we were growing up – he's eighteen months older – so when he said he was coming I thought, yes, he'd be okay. I just thought it would work. And it worked beautifully.'

An easy and effective partnership was quickly established. Don assumed responsibility for updating friends and family about Hugh's condition: fielding up to twenty incoming calls per day and ringing a list of thirty people whenever there was a major change to report. He also administered medicine, stripped beds, did washing and cooked meals. In fact, he took over all the food preparation. 'I can't eat your cooking,' he told Katherine flatly.

Don was keen on Mexican food: beans, tortillas, enchiladas, dips, sauces, small servings of meat, plenty of vegetables. He had brought his own recipe books with him. Katherine stresses what a relief it was, not to have to cook for eight weeks, before admitting to a longstanding aversion to the flavours in Mexican foods.

'It became a joke. He knew I didn't like it. But I was so grateful to him for doing the cooking that it didn't matter what he made. While I was caring for Hugh, I was so tense that I didn't ever get hungry. I only ate because my brother was there and he would tell me to sit down and have something.'

Katherine was also impressed by Don's tact, his ability to vanish when he felt the situation required it, such as when the children were visiting, or when she and Hugh needed to be alone. Hugh occasionally became very emotional about the fact that he was dying. Katherine would wrap her arms around him and they would cry together, mourning the separation that was to come.

Ministering to Hugh's body was an area where tacit embarrassment on all sides led to an unspoken division of labour. Although the children would help give their father a shower, Don did not feel comfortable about getting involved with these kinds of activities. When Hugh became bedridden, Katherine learned how to wash him by rolling him from one side to another. She also took responsibility for giving his bottom and hips an affectionate pummelling with her fingers several times each day, in order to avert bedsores.

One night in March, Katherine decided Hugh looked so dreadful that his death must be imminent. 'His whole face had collapsed and he'd gone a peculiar parchment yellow colour. His eyes were completely expressionless, it was like his brain had turned off. I really thought he was dying. I thought he was only going to last a couple of hours. I rang the children at midnight and said, "You've got to come. Please come; come now".'

Alan, Kerryn and Paul bundled spouses and offspring into cars and arrived in Armidale at five o'clock in the morning. Hugh rallied: he didn't die. When the children had gone, he explained to Katherine that she had made a mistake. Not in deciding that he was at death's door when he wasn't, but in assuming that when the time did come, he would want all his loved ones gathered around his bedside.

'Don't you dare have the family here when I die,' he told her.

'What do you mean? Of course I'm going to have them here!' Katherine said.

'Don't you dare,' Hugh reiterated. 'I'm not going to die while the family is here. You've got to promise me that you will be the only person with me when I die.'

Katherine was totally taken aback by this demand. She found it extraordinary that Hugh's sense of privacy ran so deep. She says that if she were dying, she'd want to have her bed set up in the mall in the centre of town, so everyone she knew could be there with her.

A shared sense of humour drew Katherine and Hugh together when they first met, and she feels this aspect of their relationship carried them through to the end despite all the difficulties along the way. In a letter she wrote during Hugh's final weeks, she commented that although her husband's body no longer looked like Hugh Baden, the essence of the man she had married was still alive because he could still make her laugh.

'That's such a uniting thing in a relationship, isn't it?' she says to me. 'Being able to laugh together?'

Don was amazed by Hugh's stoicism in the face of his increasing frailty and inability to look after himself. He comments that most people, given a choice, would elect to die at home in familiar surroundings, tended by their family; but he thinks that overseeing the gradual deterioration and death of a loved one takes incredible physical and mental strength. In April, he decided they couldn't continue caring for Hugh at home.

'I've wrecked my back, I can't lift him. We're going to have to send him to hospital,' he said to Katherine.

'No, no, no,' she said. 'We can make it.'

In fact, Hugh's death was only three days away. Katherine felt sure the end was near: the hallucinations of the previous night had featured Hugh repeatedly yelling out for a taxi. 'I've never heard him so agitated. "Taxi! Time to go! Come on!" I thought, he's ready to die. He's ready for out of here!'

On what turned out to be Hugh's last day, the palliative care nurse visited and told them that she didn't think it would be long now.

'But not today,' suggested Hugh.

'No, not today,' agreed the nurse.

'But maybe tomorrow?'

'Yes, maybe tomorrow.'

'Katherine thinks it's time I went, anyway,' said Hugh.

'Yes, I do,' she flashed back. They both laughed.

Hugh died that night, on the 25th of April 2006, at twelve-thirty a.m. The doctors had warned Katherine that his dying might be hard. 'They said it could be dreadful – the tumours would burst, he'd be haemorrhaging blood out of his mouth, I wouldn't be able to manage.' But in fact he died with full control and dignity, just as he had always lived. Katherine was woken from a deep sleep by a bellowed summons: 'Kath!' She leapt across the room to Hugh's bed and grabbed hold of him; he looked at her, and died.

People's names have been changed in this story

MAXINE

There are those who can reconcile themselves to death and those
who can't. Increasingly, I've come to think that it is one of the
most important ways the world divides up. Anecdotally, after all
those hours I spent in doctors' outer offices and in hospital lob-
bies, cafeterias and family rooms, my sense is that the loved ones
of desperately ill people divide the same way.

David Rieff
'Illness as more than metaphor',
New York Times, 4 December 2005

I went to the Petrea King Quest for Life Centre, that bas-
tion of positive thinking for people facing life-threatening
illness, carrying a grim secret. I had discovered that the
last-ditch treatment Mum was relying upon to save her
might succeed in stopping the spread of cancer in her
body, but there was a one in three chance that tumours

would still grow in her brain. I hadn't told her about this, reasoning that perhaps she would be in the larger, luckier category. Anyway, there was nothing she could do with the information, except worry about it. Like me.

After lunch on the first full day of the retreat, the carers met as a group to discuss their particular issues. I thought this was a forum where it might be possible to speak openly about the burden of unwanted information.

'I find it hard to stay as positive as my mother, when I know things that she doesn't know,' I said. 'Like the fact that only seven per cent of women with her advanced kind of breast cancer live for more than five years. And that thirty per cent of people taking Herceptin end up with brain tumours.'

The woman facilitating our session bristled. I was speaking the language of the enemy: gloomy scientific statistics that sap the will to survive. Quest for Life was firmly on the side of inspirational stories involving alternative therapies and miraculous remissions. The facilitator told me in no uncertain terms not to judge other people's 'journeys' or to think that the law of averages had any applicability to individuals.

'Magic happens,' she declared.

David Rieff's account of feeling impelled to fake cheery optimism as his mother, Susan Sontag, slid inexorably toward her death whilst desperately scrabbling to escape it, makes harrowing reading for those of us unable to take refuge in magical thinking. He details the extreme medical interventions Sontag insisted upon, and the gruesome physical and mental suffering they caused. He engages in self-recrimination about his own behaviour, which he sees as having been dictated by a choice that 'boiled down to hope or truth'. It is obvious that years later, he is still conflicted by his decision to endorse a struggle that he regarded as futile, and to affirm that recovery was beyond doubt when he knew death was inevitable. As a reviewer of Rieff's memoir noted, what we have here is the ultimate example of the 'bad death', the kind of miserably protracted and painful affair that overwhelms everybody with panic, guilt and bitter regrets. And afterwards, there is the pall of missed opportunities hanging over the living. The chances to interact without falsity, to speak from the heart, to say a meaningful goodbye, have all been lost.

Maxine's story is the polar opposite of David Rieff's. Her husband was utterly reconciled to the prospect of death, even when she was still reeling from the news that he had a brain tumour. She wanted to tell people about her family's experience in order to show that dying doesn't have to be fearful; it can be a serene and joyous process.

NO BIG DEAL

Maxine is a petite, attractive woman in her early fifties with brown eyes and unruly dark hair. As we sit talking at her cluttered kitchen table, light from the window over the sink catches the hennaed highlights in her curls. She is telling me how her partner, Gerard, faced his death four years ago with a cheerful acceptance that some people found confusing.

'People would ring up and ask, "How are you?" and he'd say, "I'm wonderful! I'm so good! How are you?" And they'd be totally taken aback. They'd go, "Oh ... great!" And I'd have to get on the phone and tell them, "Actually, he is still dying of a brain tumour".'

Gerard saw his death as just the end of one lifetime; a stage on the journey towards enlightenment. This understanding was rooted in almost thirty years of intensive study and dedicated practice of Buddhism. Maxine, also a longstanding Buddhist, still sounds awed by what Gerard managed to achieve when put to the test. 'He was coming from a very strong space. It was obvious nothing fazed him – he was totally at peace with whatever was going on. There was no fear. Absolutely not one scrap of fear.'

'Were you afraid?' I ask.

'I think I was annoyed with him!' she declares. We both laugh. 'He was so calm. So accepting!'

'What did you want him to do?'

'Just be a bit more emotional!' She puts her hand over her heart to indicate exaggerated sentiment. 'Like, "Oh, I'll miss you!"' She thinks for a moment, then drops back into her normal tone to add, 'Well, he was emotional, but it was about the children. He knew the attachment to them would be the hardest thing to let go of.' Sujata, the eldest daughter, mentions to me later that her father was crying when he told her how much he was going to miss seeing her and Jhana grow up.

The first indication that something was seriously wrong with Gerard was when a routine eye check revealed he had no peripheral vision. Alarmed, the optometrist recommended a brain scan. I ask Maxine about headaches, but she says there hadn't really been any symptoms. 'He'd been a bit withdrawn. I'd assumed it was because he'd just come back from a meditation retreat. He told me later that he'd been sick while he was away. He was slow, he felt like he couldn't do things properly. He thought it was his heart.'

The CT scan showed a large tumour deep inside Gerard's brain. The next day, a crowd of shocked, tearful people gathered to see Maxine and Gerard set off on the six hundred kilometre drive to Sydney for more tests. Their teenage daughters were left in the care of a friend. The car trip provided uninterrupted intimacy for intensive talking about their relationship and their life together. It was nourishing, affirming. It was also the last time Gerard was capable of having a conversation of any depth.

The couple had met at a Buddhist centre in Sydney when Maxine was twenty-three years old and Gerard was thirty-four. She was a registered nurse and he was a registered psychologist, but neither was following the conventional path for their profession. Gerard was involved in setting up a residential program offering no-drugs care for people going through major episodes of mental illness. Maxine had written to the Dalai Lama asking for a job when she finished her nursing training, and spent eight months working in a Tibetan children's village. Later, she and Gerard established a health dispensary treating Tibetan refugees with tuberculosis, at the Sera monastery in southern India.

After coming back to Australia, they tried living in various places – Tasmania, the southern highlands,

Wollongong – before finally settling on a ramshackle
property of about ten acres near the tiny town of Uralla,
in northern New South Wales. Gerard became a counsellor at the University of New England; Maxine taught yoga,
did homebirth midwifery, and worked casual shifts as a
nurse at the local hospital.

Going to Sydney for Gerard's biopsy meant a return to
close encounters with noise, traffic, pollution and crowds.
An abrupt shift to big city life can be an unwelcome side
effect of specialist treatment for country patients and their
caregivers. Maxine also had the disquieting sense that she
and Gerard were being sucked into a large, impersonal
medical machine that stripped complex identities back to
salient body parts. This patient is an eye. That one is a
brain.

In the journal she kept intermittently throughout Gerard's illness, Maxine wrote:

> Being in Sydney is horrible. Gerard is amazingly positive and
> ready for anything. Death in two weeks. Loss of speech or
> vision. Chemotherapy or radiation poisoning.

The ironic tone suggests she was finding it hard to match
Gerard's sanguine attitude. To accept his downplaying of
the situation; to agree with him that dying was no big deal.
At this point she was scared, buffeted by waves of sadness.
She wasn't sure she would be strong enough for what lay

ahead. *I don't know if I can look after a disabled husband. I
know that I am selfish and need my own space.* But she recog-
nised a spiritual opportunity in what was happening. *It's
going to be our biggest Dharma teaching yet.*

It was a few days before they were told the news that
Gerard had an inoperable glioma, an aggressive glioblas-
toma multiforme tumour, in the left parietal lobe of his
brain. Already he was deteriorating physically and mentally. *I just took Gerard for a walk and he is quite wobbly. And
his words could be a little worse today.* The prognosis was
stark: without treatment, life expectancy could be mea-
sured in terms of weeks; with treatment, months. Maxine
wrote the following poem in her journal:

Learning to overcome fear
No projecting into the future
Allow the future to be
So being left in the everpresent is all there is
Embrace life and experience without discrimination
*Easy to embrace good experience, but much harder when
things are tough & insurmountable*
Wallowing in emotional vortex is totally incapacitating
I will take on the challenge

Gerard moved into the Jean Colvin Hospital at Darling
Point while he had six weeks of radiation therapy. Jean
Colvin Hospital, operated by the charitable foundation

Can Assist, offered subsidised accommodation, meals, transport and nursing care for country people who needed to stay in Sydney for cancer treatment. Both Gerard and Maxine wanted to keep life as normal as possible for their children, so Maxine spent most of that time at home with them. She organised social activities for Gerard from a distance, putting him in touch with old friends he had not seen for ages, up to twenty years in some cases. As well as brightening his weekends, this was an opportunity for him to gather up the different strands of his past and connect them to his present situation. Another bonus was forging a stronger bond with his mother-in-law. 'My mother visited him a lot, took him out. She developed a real affection for him. And he did for her. It hadn't ever been there before.'

Maxine thinks that the enforced separation was useful for the girls as well as for her. 'It gave us time to regroup as a smaller family unit and work out what we needed to do.' One of the most urgent tasks was coming to grips with the domestic finances. This had always been Gerard's province. 'He'd done everything financially for our family. I really had very little idea. He didn't mind doing it, so I just let him. But he'd kept everything, going back years, masses of stuff. So suddenly there I was with this huge office full of papers to sort through.' There was also a large mortgage, covering the property where they lived plus a house in Armidale that Gerard had used as his consulting rooms. By the time the treatments were finished, Gerard was incapable of thinking about financial matters. Maxine got a friend to help deal with the piles of old receipts in the office and arranged to sell the Armidale house. If she tried to consult Gerard about any of it he would say, 'I don't want to know. Don't ask me that.'

Gerard came home a different man. Before, he'd spent most of his evenings locked away in the office, absorbed in his own thoughts. He had long been fascinated by the intersection between Buddhism and western psychology; he would often get up early in the morning to write down his ideas or speak them into a tape-recorder. Over the previous few years, friends and family had noticed Gerard becoming less sociable, more inclined to go off by himself. Maxine had accepted this gradual withdrawal, assuming Gerard had reached a stage of life where he felt he had to devote more energy to achieving his personal goals. Now, that introspective focus and emotional distance were gone. Gerard spent a lot of time just sitting, content to hang out with Maxine and the girls. 'There was something lovely about him that we hadn't seen before. A lot had dropped away, leaving this really childish side. He'd get enthusiastic about things. He was very present; he was living in the moment.'

I ask whether, as a Buddhist, hadn't he been like that previously? She says, 'Well, he was quite intellectual, Gerard. He always had a lot going on in terms of writing projects.'

Given that we are working together on a writing project at the moment, that comment strikes us both as highly amusing. Maxine says something that sounds like 'Watch it!' in the middle of our chortling.

Maxine and I have known each other for about fifteen years. I don't think either of us would claim the other as a close friend: more like acquaintances whose paths have intersected at certain points. She was the midwife I saw throughout my first pregnancy and she attended my labour, offering unflappable support as the planned home-birth morphed into a hospital caesarean. I knew Gerard slightly too, in his role as a counsellor at the university. My partner Chris and I saw him about commitment issues in our relationship, during our pre-babies phase. Some time later, when we had a backyard full of offspring, Gerard bought the house next door for his psychology practice. We didn't see much of him, despite the proximity. I do remember discussing pets with him once, over the fence. I was trying to offload a litter of guinea pigs; he said that his girls had 'done' guinea pigs and were on to ponies.

We had moved by the time Gerard became sick so although I heard about it, I wasn't involved at all. And then suddenly, recently, Maxine was back in my life for an intense, emotionally fraught period. She was the nurse at the other end of the phone when I rang from a conference in Canberra, desperately seeking news of my nine-year-old who had just been admitted to hospital with a burst appendix and peritonitis. Maxine had seen him come in. I wanted to hear that he was going to be fine but instead of saying reassuring things she was grave, said he looked very bad and his white blood cells were way up, or way down, I don't remember which. My son recovered, eventually. Maxine was his favourite nurse.

When I asked Maxine if she would like to be involved in my research project about home-based palliative care, she said yes, because she wanted to talk about how it was possible to bring serenity to the process of dying. At our first interview we discussed the time following Gerard's diagnosis, when the tone of the next few months was shaped by his 'no big deal' attitude; and then she told me about the period immediately after his death, when friends and family gathered to make his passing as auspicious as possible. However, this left a big hole where the middle should be, so I went back for more details.

Sujata, looking very slender in a flared handkerchief skirt and a t-shirt featuring a line of little yaks with *Yak Yak Yak* written underneath them, met me at the door and explained that her mother had gone shopping but wouldn't be long. We chatted about her recent trip to India – presumably the origin of the t-shirt – and how she was enjoying studying medicine. I was trying to be circumspect about the purpose of my visit because I didn't know what Maxine had said to her, but it turned out that Sujata knew all about it and had some memories she wanted to contribute. So the three of us sat around the kitchen table and they talked about what it was like looking after Gerard for the two months between the completion of his radiation treatment in Sydney and his death.

Despite her competency as a nurse, Maxine initially found having Gerard back home quite overwhelming. It took a few days to adjust to the fact that her husband was now a shadow of his former self, dependent on her care. The role shift was hard for the girls as well. Sujata remembers how incongruous it felt, coming home from a day at high school and having to talk her Dad through the process of using the toilet. 'He just couldn't remember how. I had to tell him to turn around and sit on it. It was little things like that that made you realise how sick he'd become. How much he'd deteriorated. Having to help him in things that you really wouldn't expect you'd ever have to.'

It was also disturbing for the family to see Gerard grappling with the frustration of not being able to express his thoughts. His mind was unravelling relentlessly. For the most part he managed to maintain his habitual even-tempered disposition, but there were occasional bouts of agitation that were all the more shocking because they were so out of character. Sujata says, 'There was one night, I'd gone to bed, but I could hear what was happening. He wanted to know something but he couldn't actually say what he wanted to know. He was very confused. He was shouting, "Maxine! Just tell me!" That was a bit scary, because he was normally so calm.'

One of Maxine's main priorities was minimising the impact of Gerard's illness on the children, so she encouraged them to continue all their usual activities. Sujata, in Year 11, was a member of the Armidale Youth Orchestra as well as playing violin and piano accordion in a popular folk music band called The Gypsy Hot Club. Jhana, in Year 8, was also a talented musician. Maxine never expected that the girls would be totally accepting of what was happening at home. She thought it was perfectly understandable that teenagers might find it annoying, or embarrassing, to have a parent around who was operating at the level of a small child, unable even to go to the toilet without assistance.

'Other families may do it differently. Other families may just stop everything and just sit around and wait for it to happen. I don't know. But it was much better for us to keep doing what we normally did. So even though at times that could have been more pressure, it was still a diversion from what was going on. Sometimes I even suggested to the girls: just stay in town, don't come home if you've got something on. Just to have a bit of space from it, because it's a really intense time,' Maxine explains.

Maxine's diversions were her work as a midwife and painting lessons at TAFE. She found the drama and joy of bringing new life into the world was therapeutic. She was relieved to discover it was actually possible to think about something other than Gerard's illness. She also felt financially driven to keep earning for as long as she could, so she would be able to take as much leave as she needed later. But I am surprised when Maxine tells me that she stayed at work until three or four weeks before Gerard died. 'Was he well enough to be left in the house by himself before then?' I ask.

'No, no, he was never on his own,' she answers. 'If I was working, we'd have someone here.'

Looking after Gerard became a community project. Friends of the family organised themselves into shifts to cover the hours Maxine would be absent. The people who came around to help were a mixture of their Buddhist friends, music friends and friends in general. They all wanted to be useful; they all wanted to spend time with Gerard. They came bearing gifts: cooked meals, fresh fruit, vegetarian quiches, special treats for Gerard like ripe strawberries and dark chocolate to dip them in. One friend gave the whole family soothing reflexology sessions during her visits.

I spoke to one of Gerard's former students, a slightly-built elderly lady with apple cheeks and soft, round, blue eyes, about her contribution during these months. As well as buying things for Gerard that she thought he would find useful, like slip-on sandals when he couldn't tie his shoe-laces, long shorts for warmer weather, and extra underwear, Beverley put her name on the roster several times a week. She would arrive about ten in the morning and spend the day sitting quietly, responding if Gerard wanted to talk or needed assistance; doing whatever was necessary in terms of preparing food, answering the phone, and washing-up; leaving when Maxine returned around six o'clock. I asked if she ever felt uncomfortable about being in their house, but she said no, she felt welcomed by the whole family and thought the dignity Gerard brought to his dying was a great teaching.

'We were just there in case he needed us, and it was very peaceful. He appreciated it very much; you felt that he really appreciated it. And he was so inspiring ... I can't remember him ever grumbling or complaining. If visitors arrived, he would always ask "How are *you?*" and focus on them. It was a privilege; we thought it was a privilege to be there,' Beverley said.

Another friend moved into the house for several weeks in October. A big, strong bikie with a shaved head and a ring through his nose, Charlie had lived with Gerard and Maxine in Wollongong. He just turned up on his motorbike and announced he'd heard Gerard was sick and he had come to help. His tattooed muscles were a welcome addition to the household. Gerard, solidly built and six feet tall, had become more tottery and Maxine and the girls were finding it hard to manage him.

With Charlie's assistance, Gerard was able to accompany Maxine, Sujata and Jhana when they went with the other Gypsy Hot Club families to Dorrigo for a music festival. Gerard was quite sick by then but didn't want to miss an opportunity to see his girls performing. Maxine remembers that he had a great time; he even came along to the pub after the main event, at midnight. 'He was just sitting there, looking a bit out of place with his beanie on and a big smile on his face. He didn't want to go to sleep. Every so often he'd really wind up and he'd want to do everything.'

The palliative care nurses came to the house once a week. Maxine knew them from the hospital and appreciated their practical attitude to managing death at home. 'They're really very good in the way that they give you permission to do what you're doing. And encourage you. It just normalises it. And anything we wanted in terms of equipment, we got the next day.' I ask what sort of aids they ended up using and Maxine and Sujata reel off a list: a special mattress that prevented bedsores by rhythmically inflating and deflating; a sheepskin for Gerard to lie on; booties for warm feet; a urodome for incontinence; a wheelchair; a lifter.

They also received supplies of medication: a low-dose morphine infuser for pain and a valium suppository in case Gerard had a seizure. When he did have a massive seizure one night, it occurred to Maxine that at this point many people would decide their loved one would be better off in hospital. 'I can see why you could panic, if you didn't have any experience and you're by yourself at four o'clock in the morning and your loved one's having a fit, you'd think: am I being unkind, keeping him at home?'

'You'd say, "I can't do this by myself. I don't want this responsibility",' I suggest.

'Or maybe, "Someone else needs to make a better medical decision about his symptoms?" But when someone's dying, it's not like you're going to be able to do anything to save them. I was just glad I had something to give him. I was pleased that I knew it was going to pass; it would probably just be short.'

Gerard's teacher, Venerable Acharya Zasep Tulku Rinpoche, came from Canada to farewell him and to help plan the practices that should be observed after his death. Maxine and Gerard had studied Gelugpa Tibetan Buddhism under Rinpoche's guidance for more than two decades. Gerard was his most advanced student; in 1995 Rinpoche had appointed him as a Dharma teacher and authorised him to give initiations.

23.10.03
Gerard is in the last throes of his life. He is succumbing to the tumour now. He has right sided weakness and cannot take

his own weight. He cannot talk. He is sleeping. He is calm. Now he doesn't have to wake for anything. He is comfortable. I am letting him go. We all have to let him go. He was incredible when Rinpoche was here. He waited for him and the day he left he let go himself. He has no attachment to life. I have deep love and attachment for him. But I can offer this to the universe. I am blessed to be going through this process with him. Now I am not working and we are full on doing palliative care. No more hope just release into the sphere of voidness and empty space.

After Rinpoche left, Gerard lapsed into semi-consciousness. He had summoned amazing resources for the visit, but crashed afterwards. 'We had a little party the last day Rinpoche was here. Gerard was sitting there on the settee, chatting away to people. You know, really making sense. Whereas in the week or two before, making sense had really come and gone... That week after Rinpoche left, he just basically went to bed.'

Friends carried Gerard out to lie in his beloved gompa, the elaborate mud-brick Tibetan Buddhist temple that Maxine and Gerard had constructed on their land soon after moving to the property. His bed was placed on the floor of a small side room. Friends and family came and went, sitting on the bed talking and laughing, as Gerard drifted in and out of consciousness, sometimes opening his eyes and smiling before sinking back into sleep. The gompa is a serene space of stained glass windows and polished wooden floors, reached by crossing a lush water garden. It does not surprise me that even with someone dying there, the atmosphere would be peaceful, not tragic. Maxine remembers one particular Sunday afternoon when Sujata and a friend were serenading Gerard on their violins, playing a mixture of classical music and Gypsy Hot Club songs. 'It was just lovely,' she says. 'So relaxing.'

24.10.03
Listening to his breath
Mattress breathing
Rhythmic air in air out
Regular timeless breath
Pulse thready bare
Thread bare
Going going gone
Gone beyond
Totally at peace
Total acceptance
No struggle
Ebb and flow of life is all around us
Letting my partner of 24 years go
I will accompany you for as long as I can then you are gone
No longer touching your living body
When you are gone
This breathing will stop

One of my friends, Trish, visited Gerard on his last day. She says he was lying on his back unconscious, occasionally quivering and moaning. Maxine increased the level of morphine he was receiving through the infuser, and asked Trish to put more salve on his stomach, where an insufficiently wrapped hot-water bottle had left a large white burn. Four people were tending to Gerard at once, trying to soothe him. Two of them were stationed at his feet, washing and massaging. Charlie began shaving his face. Trish remembers Gerard moving his head toward Charlie's hands as he worked, as though he found the touch of the warm face-cloth and the razor comforting.

Gerard Allan died at 4.30 a.m. on Tuesday 28th October, 2003. Maxine was sleeping nearby, in the main hall of the gompa, and was woken by the dogs barking. She came into Gerard's room in time to hear his final breath. She shows me a photograph of Gerard taken soon after his death. His face is peaceful. He is wearing some kind of red headgear that contrasts vividly with the bright blue pillow he is lying on, the sunny yellow bedcovering that is pulled up to his chin, and the white mosquito nets billowing softly on both sides. I comment on the beautiful arrangement of colours. She tells me that the red Tibetan hat and the yellow robe were special things that Rinpoche had given him.

The time immediately after death is highly significant in the Buddhist tradition. The spirit of the person has to be assisted to make a good karmic transition. Maxine says everything fell perfectly into place, and she felt Gerard approving all the way. Crying did occur, but mostly there was a sense of calm purposefulness. There were things to be done and a certain way to do them. The girls were swept up in the process. People were in and out of the gompa saying prayers until late at night. One of the practices involved calling out 'Hik!' while imagining the consciousness of the dead person leaving their body through the top of the head in the form of light and going into a pure land. On the second day, fourteen-year-old Jhana woke up early and was the first to go back into the gompa and resume the 'Hik!' ritual. 'I thought it was amazing, that she had the confidence to do that,' says Maxine. 'To just go in by herself with a dead body.'

A friend with woodworking skills made a simple casket out of pine board. Another communal endeavour formed around decorating the casket with brightly coloured pictures and auspicious symbols. Visitors who came to pray, stayed to paint. Maxine thinks that these practical activities in a time of heightened emotion helped to normalise the death for everyone involved. 'People were just hanging around painting the casket, having fun. My mother said she'd been nervous before she came but when she got here it was so nice, everyone was so happy.'

The funeral was harder. Although it was held at home, Maxine describes it as 'the more public' part. She felt the preceding three days had helped the family and close friends get to a point where they were ready to let Gerard go. 'But you could feel the immensity of everyone else's grief as they came to the funeral. And that was kind of hard. People are so messy with what they project onto you.' She found this irreverent. Something else she didn't like was being an object of pity. 'You get so sick of hearing the word *cope*. Like, "How are you coping, girl? How are you coping?"'

I suggest that the focus on 'coping' is shorthand for acknowledging that this could be a difficult time for her. She agrees, but says underlying people's well-meant commiseration is a mistaken view of a loved one's death as something implacably awful.

'People think it must be just horrible that it's happened, you know, that the kids have lost their father and so on. But there were so many beautiful aspects of it that the word coping doesn't seem to incorporate. What you've been through, in some ways it's the most amazing experience. You've had the privilege of going through it with someone you've loved. They've let go totally in front of you and you've been trusted to be with them. It was actually a really beautiful experience. It was transformational. It didn't feel negative at all. So I guess *cope* feels like it's really negative, and that you're having a really hard time, all the time, and you're not.'

At the funeral, no eulogies were read. In fact nothing

was said in English at all. As people came out of the rain and into the gompa, they were given a mantra to chant. THA YA THA: GATE GATE PARAGATE PARASAM-GATE BODHI SOHA. Translated, this is 'Gone, Gone, Gone Beyond, Gone Completely Beyond. Awakened. So Be It.' The mantra repetition helped ward off displays of uncontrolled emotion and preserve a calm atmosphere around the dead body. Then a group of monks arrived and took over the chanting. This was an aspect of the funeral that Maxine felt demonstrated an eerie sort of karma in operation. At the beginning of the year, long before there was any indication that Gerard was ill, they had arranged for five Tibetan monks to visit Armidale from the 25th of October to the 2nd of November, to demonstrate the art of sand mandala construction, give concerts and conduct a retreat. 'So they were here the week he died. On their day off, the monks were able to come out to the funeral and do the chanting.'

The funeral ended with Sujata and Jhana playing their violins. Then the heavy casket was loaded into the back of a station wagon and driven to the local funeral home and crematorium. Maxine had been documenting events with her camera for the past several days, but even she was surprised to find that she had taken a photo of Gerard descending into the furnace. Through a closing aperture you can see the casket sitting in a small concrete chamber, with the floor beneath it dropping like a lift. 'That's going down. He's just pressed the button. Isn't it incredible? I couldn't believe I took that photo. I don't even remember taking it.'

I comment that the funeral directors seem to have been remarkably tolerant and flexible. Allowing them to rock up with a body in a home-made coffin in the back of someone's car. Allowing the group of mourners, which included a posse of chanting monks, to go behind the scenes at the crematorium instead of insisting that they all stay on the conventional side of the discreet black curtain. 'Oh, Piddington's were fantastic!' says Maxine. She tells me that home-death, like home-birth, is all about empowering yourself to take control of the process rather than being passively swept along by the system. Ensuring that Gerard had the sort of death he wanted, the full Buddhist send-off, was the highest gift, the last act of love, that she could give to him.

15.11.03

I am learning to function and find a way to be clear despite overwhelming emotions. Last night was hard, coming home to an empty house. The girls had symphony practice and I stayed at home and felt lonely and sorry for myself. But tonight has been better. I felt anxious about being alone again and was going to ring someone but after going for a walk I started enjoying myself. Enjoying being alone. Noting that emotions, thoughts, feelings, sensations all pass. That's what I told Sujata. Everything passes. Take refuge. Dharma is all that truly helps. Everything else gives temporary relief. Even people.

KAYE

The picture that emerges from the public submissions is that carers for dying people 'make do' with whatever information and
support is available to them or comes to their attention, should
they happen to be at the right place and at the right time, or have
the know-how to navigate the system.

'The hardest thing we have ever done': Full Report
of the national inquiry into the social impact of
caring for terminally ill people,
Palliative Care Australia, 2004, p. 8

My Aunty Caroline was leaving the palliative care unit,
after a meeting where she had committed to nursing her
terminally-ill sister at home, when a staff member said
offhandedly, 'Is there anything you'd like?'

'Oh, a hospital bed, a nurse, some money,' Caroline
laughed.

'Well, we might be able to manage the hospital bed.'

In this casual manner we received an indispensable piece of equipment for nursing my mother. With the touch of a button we could change Mum's position from lying to sitting, an operation she was unable to perform herself. Other buttons directed the whole bed to rise higher, sparing our backs as we rolled our patient from side to side; or to sink lower, making it easier to get her in and out of bed.

The 'lifter' we received later came in a similarly serendipitous fashion. I would never have thought to enquire if such a thing might be available if my mother-in-law, who has a nursing background, had not raised it as a possibility. She said that with a lifter, one carer could manage the transfers from the bed to the wheelchair, instead of two people being needed. When I asked, I was told that yes, we could put our name down for a lifter, and in due course, one arrived.

You could be forgiven for concluding that the resources for home-based palliative care are rationed on a guess-what-we've-got basis.

During my interview with Kaye Ambrose, I was astounded to hear that eight weeks before her husband died, she'd had to arrange access to palliative care services herself; even though John's death from prostate cancer was long expected, and despite the fact that for six months she'd been telling anyone who would listen that he was suffering from constant nausea.

'You weren't referred to palliative care, not even for symptom control, you had to go looking for them yourself?' I ask, thinking I must have misunderstood what she had just said.

'That's right,' she replies. 'And when I contacted them, they couldn't believe that neither the oncologist nor the GP had ever suggested getting palliative care. They told me palliative care should be brought in at the beginning, when the diagnosis is made, not towards the end like I'd assumed. That's why I contacted them. Because he was going downhill and I knew the time was coming when I needed that help to care for him at home. So I downloaded a form from the internet and sent it in.'

STAYING HAPPY

Ten years before he died, John Ambrose was told he had only five years to live. He had smiled and joked his way through the ups and downs of prostate cancer for so long that his wife didn't know how to break the news that he wasn't going to bounce back this time. A palliative care social worker had suggested Kaye stop work immediately if she wanted to be home for John's final weeks. Kaye was a teacher at Swinburne TAFE and a new term had just begun. She knew telling her husband she was taking leave was tantamount to announcing his death was imminent, so she said she was home because her students were on work experience.

John and Kaye first met in 1963, when she was almost nineteen and he was twenty-four. They were both members of the Williamstown Light Opera Company in Melbourne.

Kaye had studied music and ballet and loved singing and dancing; John was musically untrained but had a glorious Irish tenor voice. On their first date, a ninetieth birthday party for one of John's great-aunts, John said so frequently 'I'd like you to meet my sister,' that by the time the fifth female was introduced in this manner, Kaye had decided he must be having her on. She hadn't known he was the only boy in a large Catholic family.

The divide between Catholics and Protestants was strong in those days and both Kaye and John were heavily involved in their respective churches. They broke off their relationship several times, thinking religious differences made it futile to continue. When they eventually married in 1966 it was because John had decided his spiritual needs could be met outside Catholicism. His parents were appalled by his defection. The wedding service was held at Kaye's Methodist church in Essendon; John's mother and four of his sisters came but refused to enter the church for the ceremony; his father stayed at home with the other sister.

The newlyweds went to live in the affordable outer suburb of Wantirna South, near the Dandenong Ranges. John had qualified as a painter and decorator but was working as a sales representative for a wholesale stationery and art supplies company. Kaye was teaching office administration subjects at a business college. They both joined the local Methodist church and sang in its choir; they were too far from Williamstown to continue with the opera company. On their occasional visits to John's parents in Newport, his father completely ignored them: he would not eat at the same table; he would not sit in the same room. Finally, one Christmas, after Kaye had greeted her father-in-law with a kiss, as she always did whether he liked it or not, he broke four years of silence to express regret at the recent loss of her first baby, a girl who died two days after birth. From that point, all animosities faded away. John and Kaye's second daughter, Robyn, was born in 1970, followed by a son, Steven, three years later. Both grandparents died when the children were little and three of John's sisters also chose to 'marry out', so the next generation grew up unaware that religion had ever been a source of contention within the family.

I came into contact with Kaye Ambrose through a fellow postgraduate student, Siobhan McHugh, who was researching mixed marriages in Australia. John had died at home a few months before Siobhan interviewed Kaye, so the story of how bitterly his parents had opposed his union with a non-Catholic was particularly poignant given that Kaye had lovingly nursed him to the end of forty years together. On being told about this project, Kaye agreed to participate in my research as well. Siobhan shared the section of her audio recording relating to John's last weeks and Kaye spoke to me on the phone and sent me eulogies, diary notes, biographical material and photographs.

From all this information, a picture emerged of John: a big man who stood six feet high and weighed more than sixteen stone; a sports fanatic who excelled at golf and watched the football on two television sets at once; a clown whose wit and tomfoolery could reduce his family to tears of hysterical laughter even in a restaurant; an animal lover who delighted in pets of all kinds and called every one of them 'pal'; a keen home handyman and gardener; and, of course, a singer who performed in choirs until a year before he died. His daughter Robyn wrote about him as:

The dad who enjoyed playing Santa by scattering straw everywhere each Christmas, and reinforced Mum with a firm voice when we were playing up to her, and brought us gifts each time he was away for work, and let us draw on the side of the house in permanent marker, and made our school dress-up costumes, and tinkered with home-made fizzy drinks, and brought home the latest and brightest technology (go Beta video!) and most surprisingly accepted that I brought a motorcycle gang home and befriended them all;

The husband who totally, constantly and romantically loved our mother, and admired, affectionately joked with and supported her without compromising her independence for over forty years;

The grandfather who lovingly held and gently whispered to his grandchildren after they were born and set about being the sweetest, funniest, kindest, most loving papa in the world.

John was diagnosed with inoperable prostate cancer in July 1997, just before his fifty-eighth birthday. There had been no indication that anything was amiss – apart from him needing to get up more often at night to urinate, something he had assumed was due to age – until a routine health check revealed an enlarged prostate. Kaye went to a specialist with him to get the results of further tests. The urologist reported that the prostate specific antigen (PSA) reading of 45 was right off the scale, indicating cancer, and informed them that John had about five years to live. He delivered the news, says Kaye, 'with as much feeling, empathy and understanding as if he were telling us our car had something wrong.'

The death sentence was so unexpected that it left them feeling numb for several months. Initially, John did not want anyone else to know: he didn't want people feeling sorry for him or making a fuss over him. Kaye says she found it hard to express her own compassion in a way that wouldn't be interpreted as 'fussing'. She would often look at John as he slept in front of the television and feel great pity and helplessness, knowing there was nothing she could do to take the burden from him. She did convince John to allow her to tell their close friends and family about the diagnosis. The only people John spoke to himself were three of his closest mates, men he had grown up with. For twenty years they had met as a group every six months; he told them the news one evening when they came to his home for dinner with their wives.

Within a week of seeing the urologist, John had registered with the Anti-Cancer Council and joined a prostate cancer support group. He attended their monthly meetings for two years, until he felt there was nothing more he could learn about the disease and its treatments. He continued to take phone calls from newly-diagnosed men as they were referred to him, invariably seeking to bolster their confidence by describing how well he was going. He was having regular injections of the testosterone-inhibiting hormone, Zoladex, which causes impotence, but his way of dealing with this side-effect was to make jokes about it. Kaye notes that she and the children observed that without testosterone, John seemed to be a kinder, quieter person – less aggressive, more patient. I ask if he had noticed the change himself, and she replies that he never spoke about it.

After five years of Zoladex, John's PSA readings began to climb again. The urologist said this meant the cancer was no longer responding to the hormone treatment and referred him to an oncologist. Kaye had to explain to John that an oncologist was a specialist in cancer diagnosis and treatment. Scans showed the disease was progressing into the bones. At this stage John was still employed full-time as the manager of a sheltered workshop, having been retrenched from his previous position as a salesman. He used to tell Kaye he would never complain about health problems after seeing the bravery his disabled clients brought to their daily lives. Despite the fatigue caused by his cancer, he remained an active member of the Hilltop Singers. Kaye says: 'He would come home from work absolutely exhausted, fall asleep over the tea table and drag himself off for the evening's choir practice.'

Gradually the cancer began to encroach upon John's capacity to carry on with life as normal. He collapsed playing golf one day and had to concede that he no longer had the stamina required to walk around the course. The family discussed buying him an electric buggy but could not afford to do more than rent one occasionally. John also began to suffer from muscular soreness as his bones became weaker. His work in the storeroom at Scope required him to lift and carry things, and as the only man in the local Hilltop Singers he felt obliged to help wheel the rehearsal piano from one room to another each week.

'That was something he should never have been doing,' says Kaye. 'We all said to him: "John, you're not to move the piano." But his pride wouldn't let him stand by and watch while the women did it.'

John persisted with such physically demanding tasks despite the fact that they often resulted in spasms of pain later. Kaye attributes this refusal to acknowledge constraints to a 'typical aussie male ego' and says that John only ever spoke about having 'muscle problems' – the sort of thing he'd had in the past from playing sport – and never related these symptoms to his cancer. She didn't challenge his reasoning: 'I thought, well, if he's happy with that, why say anything different?'

Toward the end of 2003, the oncologist decided to try John on a bone-strengthening drug called Zometa. After having the second monthly treatment, John began vomiting on his way to work; within a few days he was in the renal ward of St Vincent's Public Hospital on the verge of kidney failure. He responded well to plasma exchange treatments and was eager to come home for Christmas. Kaye was less enthusiastic. John hadn't eaten for twelve days; he was weak and exhausted and still shaking from an adverse reaction to a component of the donated blood. 'I was dead against him being discharged because I felt he was too big a responsibility for me,' recalls Kaye. 'But the hospital said John could go on Christmas Eve if he wanted to, so I took him home. He had a restless night and wasn't interested in eating the next day. He had a few drinks, took a photo of me, and then went back to bed. So my Christmas lunch was eaten alone watching the TV.'

Over the next week, Kaye took John back to St Vincent's hospital every second day for more infusions of plasma and calcium. It was a two hour round trip into the city and each treatment lasted seven hours, so she filled in the time by wandering around shops and going to the cinema. Blood tests on the 5th of January showed John's kidney function had returned to normal, but it took three months for him to regain enough strength to go back to work.

In August 2004, John underwent his first radiotherapy treatment to relieve the constant pain in his pelvic area. To Kaye's surprise and relief, the treatment worked so well that they were able to go on the touring holiday of New Zealand that she had booked for September, instead of having to cancel it. John even managed to play two rounds of golf while he was there.

For most of their married life, John had claimed to be uninterested in overseas travel. Kaye was the opposite: she had wanted to go overseas from when she was fifteen. The opportunity had finally arisen in 1989, when she was forty-five: the children were in their late teens, old enough to be left behind, and both Kaye and John had long-service leave owing to them. But when Kaye had suggested going to Europe, John had replied he couldn't see the point of spending so much money to look at old ruins. So she went off on a guided tour without him and returned seven weeks later with twenty-five new friends who met regularly thereafter to swap reminiscences about their fabulous experiences. Kaye thinks this might have piqued John's interest, because when she raised the issue of travel again, in 2001, he announced that he'd quite like to see Canada. They went with another couple and had a cruise to Alaska and a stopover in Hawaii as well. From then on, John was hooked: 'You couldn't keep him out of a travel agency,' says Kaye.

Early in 2005, the oncologist advised John to give up work before starting a series of chemotherapy treatments aimed at slowing the progress of the cancer. By this stage, the number of days John was calling in sick were almost equal to the number he was able to attend work, so he retired in April. The chemotherapy was a mild dose and at the end of it, John felt well enough to do more travelling. During the TAFE break in September, he and Kaye went to Denmark for ten days to stay with old friends. Their Danish hosts were a doctor and a nurse and so managed to set an appropriate pace whilst showing off their country. Kaye notes that John, the 'old ruins' sceptic, was awestruck by the fifteenth century architecture. On their return from Denmark, they had two days to recover from jetlag before setting off again, this time on a cruise to Noumea with Kaye's brother and his wife.

Although John was retired, Kaye was still employed full-time as a TAFE teacher. She says John enjoyed being at home at first: he shopped and cooked dinner and pottered about in the garden, but he found it frustrating when he no longer had the energy to do much. 'He got to the point where he couldn't manage jobs in the garden or around the house. There were things that needed fixing but he didn't have the strength to do them. And there's only so much television you can watch in a day.'

Recognising that his father was becoming depressed, Steven and his partner Tessa dropped in one day bearing two irresistible sources of diversion and company: a grey and white male kitten that John called Zorro and a ginger and white female that Kaye named Tosca.

In October 2006, John and Kaye celebrated their forti-eth wedding anniversary with a party and a trip to Perth. John had a temporary surge in his energy levels; he thor-oughly enjoyed the week in Perth and even managed to outwalk Kaye during their sightseeing. However, he had begun feeling less interested in eating and was losing weight; this was the start of a slide that would take him from obese to gaunt in the course of the next eight months.

'John was feeling nauseous and had trouble keeping any food or medicine down,' says Kaye. 'Each morning I would go off to work feeling guilty for leaving him sitting on the edge of the bed dry-retching. He spent most of the time sleeping. I'd come home at four o'clock and he wouldn't have eaten anything since I left.'

Swinburne TAFE was only a five minute drive from where they lived. Kaye would ring regularly to check on John. When he stopped bothering to answer the phone, she began coming home during breaks; finally she was only going to work when she had a class to teach. She says having a sympathetic, understanding manager made this possible.

When teaching finished in mid-December 2006, John began a week of radiotherapy treatments on his back and shoulder. Kaye found getting him to the early morning appointments in the city a stressful process: driving through peak hour traffic to the hospital, stopping out the front and running to find a wheelchair because John was too weak to walk, leaving him waiting in the foyer while she drove around trying to find a parking spot. She felt at her wit's end because no-one seemed to be listening to the fact that John was constantly nauseated and not eating. He complained that it felt like he had a fur-ball in his throat. They'd asked the oncologist about it, and he'd patronisingly suggested they go to a GP as it was nothing to do with the cancer; they'd mentioned it to the radiotherapist, and they'd been to see John's GP three times and Kaye's GP once. The only solution they were offered was anti-nausea tablets and John couldn't keep those down. Kaye finally decided she had to take action.

'The day after radiotherapy treatments finished I took him to our local public hospital and insisted that he had to be admitted and treated. I told them I didn't care if it was Christmas. While we were in the emergency department waiting to be attended to, John broke down and cried for the first time since his diagnosis. They booked him into a private hospital and he spent the next sixteen days there with a very bad infection. When I went in on the morning of Christmas Eve he was crying and when I went in on Christmas Day he was crying again. He had two tests, a gastroscopy and a barium swallowing test, but nothing showed up in his throat.'

John came home from hospital in early January 2007 slightly better but the nausea, lack of appetite and exhaustion continued. Steven and Tessa had arranged to marry on the 18th of February and very much wanted John to be at the wedding. Kaye says, 'He wouldn't have missed it for the world. He summoned all his strength to be there even though it was a forty degree day. He was determined to have a dance with each of his five sisters, myself, Robyn, Tessa, and her mother Helen.' John managed every dance he had promised and then spent the next few weeks recovering.

In April 2007, Kaye registered John for palliative care by searching on the internet, downloading a form, and sending it in. The palliative care nurses were amazed to hear that not one of the doctors dealing with John's case had ever thought to mention the home-based services available for terminally ill people and their families. It was an enormous relief for Kaye to know that nurses would visit regularly and she would have a phone number she could use, twenty-four hours a day, seven days a week, to get practical help and advice. However, John didn't understand the importance of this at first. 'Oh, I don't need them,' he said, when Kaye asked if he would agree to the palliative care nurses coming to the house.

'But I do,' Kaye pointed out.

In John's final months, Kaye was very glad to have the palliative care nurses on hand: suggesting medication to ease discomfort, liaising with doctors and hospitals, and helping to organise emergency appointments. Above all else, she appreciated the compassionate, personalised support they offered to both carer and patient, as she had found this to be a quality noticeably absent in almost all their interactions with the medical system.

John went to hospital so frequently that Kaye eventually compiled a dossier of all his medications and his previous admissions and discharge documents, in order to avoid having to recite the same details over and over. 'You get asked the same set of questions by the guys in the ambulance, by the nurse at the hospital, and by the doctor on duty. So I had everything in writing and I could just hand it to them.'

'Wasn't it all in the hospital records?' I ask.

'Course it was!' she says. 'But they didn't look it up. Every different doctor and nurse that you get, you start from scratch again.'

Chemotherapy had caused John's lower teeth to decay and his oncologist had been urging him for a year to have them extracted. John already wore a plate for his top teeth but he had delayed having treatment for the bottom ones, wanting to spare Kaye the expense. Finally they became so infected that they had to be taken out. Kaye remembers this vividly, not only because it was the starting point for a sequence of medical complications, but because it illustrated the robustness of John's sense of humour. After all his remaining teeth had been extracted and he was sitting in the dentist's chair with his mouth stuffed full of gauze, unable to talk, John motioned to Kaye for pen and paper. He wrote: 'I've changed my mind.'

The next day, when his gums began to bleed uncontrollably, John rang Kaye at work and got her to take him back to the dentist. The dentist tried glue and then stitching but she couldn't stop the bleeding. After persisting for three hours she called an ambulance, and John was taken to Monash Medical Centre where an oral surgeon spent another three hours stitching his gums at a deeper level until the bleeding finally stopped. By then it was eight p.m. and they were told John needed to stay in hospital under observation. Kaye was worried about him not having any pyjamas or toiletries. 'I haven't brought anything for you to stay overnight,' she said.

'Not even a toothbrush?' John quipped.

John came home from hospital with diarrhoea due to an allergic reaction to the antibiotics in his drip. Lomotil tablets fixed that, but a few days later he developed thrush and a blockage in his bladder. Kaye rang the local medical clinic that she and John had attended for decades but was told they didn't make house calls. An ambulance took John to a local private hospital where, says Kaye, 'An insensitive, not very gentle doctor inserted a catheter, drained the urine, and said I could bring him back if the problem recurred.' It did recur, the next day. John was apprehensive about a repeat episode of the pain. The palliative care nurses booked an ambulance to take him to the local public hospital this time and arranged for him to be seen on arrival. The doctor there was careful and kind; he re-inserted the catheter and advised that it be left in place.

Kaye got on the phone to the medical clinic and told them their service wasn't good enough. Her own GP, who was a partner in the practice, agreed to take John as a patient and visit him at home.

The following week, John was back to hospital again because he'd been bleeding into the catheter bag. He was given three units of blood and a vitamin K injection and discharged the next day. Test results were sent to his oncologist. John was due to see the oncologist several days later, on the 7th of May, but the ambulance failed to pick him up for the appointment. Kaye contacted the oncologist's office and found no arrangements for an ambulance had been made. That afternoon the oncologist's nurse rang her back with a stark explanation: 'Terry has all the blood test results and doesn't need to see John again because there's nothing more he can do for him.'

The family support officer from palliative care visited and spoke to Kaye about John's deterioration. 'I asked her when she thought I should give up work,' recalls Kaye. The woman replied she was not supposed to offer advice about that, but when Kaye pressed for an answer, she said, 'If I were you, and I wanted time with him, then I'd stop now.'

Kaye immediately arranged to take leave but did not tell John about it straight away: 'I thought – if I say I'm home permanently now, he'll know that's the end for him. So initially I said to him that I was home for a couple of weeks because my students were on work experience. Then I spoke to the social worker again. I said, "The big problem is that everyone's pussyfooting around at the moment. We don't know what John's thinking. We don't know how much he knows." And she said, "All you can do is broach the issue and see if he'll talk about it".'

Several days later, when John was obviously feeling exasperated by the nausea and vomiting that had afflicted him for months, Kaye raised the issue of his impending death. John evinced no surprise; he said he'd known ten years ago that the prostate cancer would get him eventually. He added that he was feeling very tired of everything. 'I asked him if he was frightened; he said he wasn't but he didn't know what would happen. I said, "All I know is that you'll probably sleep more and be awake less." I knew some other things that palliative care had told me but I didn't pass those on to him.'

Kaye and John did not discuss the matter any further. However, a week later he told her about a dream. In it, he was driving to the local hospital at ten kilometres per hour and everyone on the road was abusing him for going so slowly. He got to the emergency department, parked the car, turned off the ignition, and then had a heart attack and died.

'I didn't know how to react,' Kaye tells me. 'I just said something silly: "I hope you didn't crash my car!" Even though I could see the symbolism so clearly – his illness was dragging on and he was taking so long to die: he felt he was a burden on other people. It was time to turn everything off and finish it. I told the palliative care social worker about the dream later and she said it was quite a revelation.'

The palliative care nurses were finding it difficult to give John sponge baths and change his catheter bag because the bed he shared with Kaye was too low. They offered to arrange delivery of a hospital bed with a pressure-relieving mattress. John said no, he didn't need a hospital bed. Kaye explained it was an occupational health and safety issue and suggested if the hospital bed were put in the lounge room, he could just move into it when the nurses were due to come. John agreed to this arrangement and it worked for a couple of weeks.

'Initially he could walk between the beds, then I had to help him, then he used a walking frame that had belonged to my father, then he couldn't do that anymore so I got a computer chair with castors and brought him in that way. Eventually he was too weak to get from one room to the other so he stayed in the hospital bed all the time.'

Kaye says that right to the end, John retained the capacity to joke about his condition. She knew he felt sensitive about his appearance – basically he was like a skeleton with skin on – so when her boss from TAFE, the one who had been so understanding about Kaye's role as a carer, asked if she could visit, Kaye checked to see if John minded. 'He said, "No – but I'd better look sick, hadn't I?"'

One of the services palliative care arranged for bed-bound patients was regular massages. During a long relaxing session with his masseuse, John mentioned that he was waking up at four a.m. with a lot going through his mind. He agreed it would be good to talk to the palliative care social worker about this. Kaye thought, 'Great! He's finally going to speak to someone about his feelings.' However, by the time the social worker came two days later, John was no longer able to talk. She spoke to him, and he indicated that he heard her by squeezing her hand, but he could not tell her what had been worrying him.

Meanwhile, Kaye and John's daughter Robyn had been attempting to deal with her own emotional torment by writing down the anguish she felt unable to share with her beloved father.

This is horrible – I can't switch off my brain. All day long, pictures past and present randomly flash into my mind until I feel like I can't see anything else. I look at something and I see Dad ... looking pained and fragile, trying to keep his chin up and be brave for us ... I see the haunted fear in his eyes and pray I'm keeping up a good enough act that he can't see that reflected in mine ... and then reality snaps into sharp focus.

There is a sickly knot in my stomach that keeps churning around – every now and then it rises up to give me heartburn and asthma, other times it sinks and I feel a revolted urge to throw up. I have a constant knot in my throat that keeps threatening to choke me, and occasionally it does. Then the tear ducts get in on the act and I feel like I'm falling apart at the seams.

My world is. My father is.

How can I sit by nonchalantly and have subconscious bets with myself about how and when the inevitable will strike?

How can I sit by making jokes to 'cheer him up'?

How do any of us prepare for this?

How can he not be thinking about his fate – if I can't stop I'm sure he's doing the same thing ... only for him, it's so much worse.

How do I deal with the selfishness of worrying about what effect this will have on <u>my</u> life?

What must it be like to spend each day wondering if you're about to experience excruciating pain, or to hope each time you go to bed that you will wake up again ... or that you won't?

In 'Reflections', Robyn vividly and lovingly depicts John as a person, and all that he meant to her, concluding with: 'I love my daddy with the same awe and wonderment as I always have – a part of me will always see him through the eyes of a five-year-old. He's my hero, my superman, and I don't want to lose him ... '

On the morning of the social worker's visit, Kaye showed her what Robyn had written, saying, 'It's such a pity John doesn't know about it.'

'You could always read it to him,' the social worker suggested.

Later that afternoon, when she was alone with John, Kaye did so. John listened with his eyes closed. When she finished reading, Kaye asked him, 'Did you hear that?' John nodded, yes. Three hours later he was in a coma. Kaye, Robyn and Steven sat with him that night. Two palliative care nurses came the next morning to move him into a more comfortable position, and the GP visited at lunchtime. Kaye showed the doctor to the front door and then went back to John. He had died whilst she was out of the room, at one p.m. on the 22nd of June, 2007.

BEN

Guilt comes no matter what you have or haven't done. To live without guilt after the death of a loved one, a person would have to accede to literally everything the other person wanted. And what that means is living one's entire life in attendance of the other's death ...

David Rieff

Swimming in a Sea of Death: A son's memoir, 2008, p. 99

Love and resentment, togetherness and mystifying disconnection, personal tragedy and domestic politics ... This was a gruelling story to write, because it roused a welter of conflicting emotions in me. As a mother and a feminist, I felt great empathy and compassion for Lynne, a woman with three small children, who died before she could work out how to satisfy the part of her unfulfilled by childrearing and domestic duties. However, it was Ben's version of their family life that I was portraying, and I also sympathised with his impatience at Lynne's indecisiveness, and identified with his drive to shine in his chosen profession. Also, I could understand the threads of ambivalence, confusion and guilt woven through his account of the loving attachment he and Lynne had shared. In the self-justifications and self-doubts he expressed, I could see echoes of my own concerns about whether I had proved a good daughter to my mother.

This story provokes strong responses in readers, too. A close friend of both Ben and Lynne raised the question of whether it was fair to confront the couple's children with the 'failings' of their mother:

> *Failings that we all have. Failings that are overlooked with the passage of time, or forgotten as they have been redeemed by subsequent actions. Devastatingly, Lynne will never be given this opportunity.*

I think the failings are evenly distributed in this story, and one day Chloe, Nick and Luke will be old enough to read it and accept the simple truth that adults are flawed and parenting small children can be demanding and difficult. The real tragedy of this story lies in the timing. You can't help feeling that everything would have become easier, given time.

THREE STEPS
BEHIND

I remember Ben as the gregarious and self-assured young man who baffled our group by asking where he could get hold of a list of every emotion a person could experience. Armed with such a list, he thought he might be able to articulate the mix of feelings that had been roiling around inside him during the months of his wife's illness. Thinking about the oddness of this request now, I try to put a name to what it evoked in me then: and come up with wry compassion.

It was August 2004, the first full day of the five we would spend together at the Quest for Life centre in the Southern Highlands town of Bundanoon. Twenty-two people of mixed ages occupied a motley assortment of chairs arranged in a large circle. Irrespective of whether they were perching straight-backed on a firm chair or sinking deeply into a plush one, everybody looked tense. More than half the people there had cancer or some other form of life-threatening disease. Interspersed between the unwell were the significant others: lovers, mothers, spouses, siblings, adult children, friends. We knew this session, 'Stories from Participants', was going to be a confronting one. In recounting our tragic tales we would be bringing out the demons: the suppressed fears, the half-acknowledged griefs, the too-tentative hopes.

The egalitarian arrangement of chairs did not stop the circle from having a dominant point. It was where Petrea was sitting. Petrea King is one of Australia's most famous cancer survivors, and a purveyor of hope, self-help strategies and inspirational messages to those embarking on their own journeys into the territory of serious illness. Not 'terminal' illness, Petrea had stipulated in her beautifully modulated voice, smiling her glorious crescent moon smile, during our orientation session the previous afternoon. She argued that the word terminal should never be applied to people. 'Terminals are for buses, trains, and computers,' she said.

Nevertheless, when it was time for Lynne, Ben's partner, to tell her story, she was clear-eyed about the prognosis that had brought her there. She said she was thirty-four years old, her children Chloe, Nick and Luke were aged five, three and one, and she had terminal ovarian cancer. She matter-of-factly chronicled the cysts and tumours that had bedeviled her pregnancies and the surgeries and chemotherapy that had failed to halt the cancer's progress. The calmness of her delivery was typical of the cohort of patients in the room that day. The stories that were told were harrowing, brave, sad, funny, desperate, inspiring and confronting; but it was the support people who broke down, who struggled to remain articulate as they described the experience of standing by while someone they loved was put through the wringer. My mother spoke before me and told her story with composure; my first sentence ended with tears and a battle to secure my voice. I understood why Ben might feel such bewilderment that he could think working through a list of emotions would help him sort out his feelings.

I already knew a bit about Lynne and Ben because I had met them the night before when they checked into our four-bedroom lodge. After dinner, six of us had sat chatting over hot drinks in the shared central lounge/kitchen area. Lynne had been a quiet presence on the edge of the conversation but she seemed to be in good spirits, occasionally volunteering an insightful or funny comment. Ben was the sort of fellow who teases strangers, even grey-haired ones, with ease. 'That's very precise, Pat,' he had said to my mother, when she regaled us with some obscure biographical detail about the other Australian cancer-survival guru, Ian Gawler.

I'd encountered Ben again before breakfast on the day of the 'Stories from Participants' session, at nearby Morton National Park. I'd been scanning the walks featured on a noticeboard near the entrance when Ben came along at a fast jog. He told me he hadn't exercised for a long time; he used to be very fit when he played rugby and he wanted to get back into shape. He looked okay to me, but rather lightly built for a footballer.

Over the next few days our early morning exercise routines merged into a joint activity. Ben slowed his pace to my brisk walk and we talked non-stop as we strode along shady bush tracks and puffed up steep hills. I learned that although he was now spending most of his time at home with Lynne and the children, before that he'd been something of a rising star in his profession as a pharmacist. He had served on a government committee investigating online health initiatives; the pharmacy he part-owned in Forster-Tuncurry was the biggest in the district, employing over thirty people; and two years earlier it had won an Australia-wide medal of excellence in pharmacy practice. Ben now wanted to sell his share of the pharmacy so he could focus on being with his family, but his business partner was being unhelpful and the process had become mired in correspondence between solicitors. He also spoke about how he wanted Lynne to be happy in whatever time she had left to her, but felt that he was always three steps behind in figuring out how she was feeling and what she needed from him. He said despite his best intentions, he never seemed to be able to satisfy her. If he washed the kitchen floor before going to work, he would be told he should have done the dishes instead. If he stepped back because she seemed to be having a good morning and she was keen to do something independently, he would get roused on in the afternoon for not helping out enough.

I lent a sympathetic ear to these concerns and tried to reassure Ben that what he was describing sounded quite normal given the stresses of their situation. To an outsider, they appeared to be a close, happy couple. At the time, I didn't realise I was seeing the relationship at a high point. Being temporarily freed from the pressures and distractions of tending to small children, and feeling nourished and uplifted by the retreat, had combined to create a sense of harmony that had not really been typical of their life together in recent years. In fact, only a month earlier Lynne had wondered yet again whether they should split up.

'What were you looking for, at the Petrea King retreat?' I ask Ben, several years later. We are sitting on the back verandah of his home near Forster, on the north coast of New South Wales. Trawling a Cancer Council web site earlier that year, I had found an article he'd written that told me Lynne had died at the end of 2004. I tracked down his address and sent him a letter, with belated condolences, and an invitation to participate in this project.

I asked about the motivation for going on the Quest for Life program because it had been my impression that many people – my mother included – went along to Bundanoon hoping to get the secret of how to survive cancer straight from the horse's mouth. This was despite the fact that Petrea stresses, both during the program and in the book of the same name, that her focus is more about the quality of the life lived than its duration:

> Many people come to me looking for the rosy path to healing. They want to be told all the things which they must do in order to heal themselves of their disease. Many do not want to hear about the thorns; the anguish, fears, angers, resentments, guilts and shames, the unresolved relationships which need to be addressed in order to truly heal their lives ... I've known many who died 'healed' and this accomplishment is every bit as miraculous and wondrous as those who healed and continued to stay in their bodies ... We don't value a life by its length. It's not how long we live which is of importance. It's the spirit with which we live that will continue to nourish the hearts of those who knew us.
>
> Petrea King, *Quest for Life* 2004, p. 46

Lynne went to Bundanoon looking for peace of mind in whatever time she had remaining to her. Whether or not she succeeded in healing her life, she didn't continue to stay in her body; in fact, she died four months after attending the Quest for Life program. What I can glean of the thorns she needed to address, the healing she managed to achieve, the spirit she brought to her living and to her dying, and the impact all of this had upon those who loved her and who cared for her, rests primarily on the candid account Ben gave me of their years together, plus a small amount of writing Lynne did during her final months.

'What was I looking for at Petrea King's place?' Ben echoes. 'I'll tell you what I wanted. That Lynne got a bit of happiness and wasn't cranky with me, and with life in general.'

Ben and Lynne first met playing football. Even though she wasn't particularly sporty, Lynne joined a mixed touch footy team in 1995. By the end of the season the team had won the grand final and team-mates Ben and Lynne had become a couple. She was twenty-five, living in Manly, and working for a large insurance company; he was twenty-two, living at home with his adoptive parents in Roseville, and doing his graduate year as a pharmacist. Part of their connection was that they had each spent time overseas when they finished school and could swap reminiscences about the places they had seen. Ben had gone to England on a football scholarship in 1991 and made forays into Europe, Canada, the United States and Mexico. Lynne had spent all of 1990 and 1991 travelling in Britain, Europe, Asia and the United States, supporting herself with occasional bar-jobs and working as a nanny. Fourteen years later, in the handcrafted book in which she was recording her memories for her children, she recalls with transparent relish her time as an intrepid world-wanderer:

> *Apart from having 3 children, the most exciting thing I've ever done was spend 2 years travelling overseas living out of a backpack. I spent some of the time living and working in the US but mostly I travelled. I went to Ireland, Scotland, France (twice), Italy, Austria (twice), Germany, Hungary, Czechoslovakia (twice), Portugal, Switzerland, Greece, Turkey, Egypt, India, Bali, Thailand – oh and I almost forgot Holland and Belgium.*
>
> *I had many many adventures – I did lots of treks, some on camels, some on elephants, some on donkeys and some on foot. I climbed mountains, swam in beautiful oceans, slept on glorious beaches, slept in dodgy train stations, hitchhiked, took drugs, saw amazing architecture, met wonderful people, met weird people.*
>
> *Had an amazing exciting time.*

Lynne came back from overseas and resumed her work as an insurance underwriter. It was just a job, a way to earn money; it was not something she found intrinsically satisfying. Before she left school she had wanted to be an airhostess, but her parents had dissuaded her, saying the finance industry offered more stable prospects. Later she often expressed regret about not having followed her original inclination.

Ben's habit of setting clear goals for himself and striving hard to achieve them was in marked contrast to Lynne's more *laissez faire* approach to life. He had considered other healthcare career options – veterinary science, medicine, physiotherapy – but having ended up in pharmacy he focused his ambitions on success in that profession. He split his year of work experience between two leading pharmacies: one was innovative in its dealings with customers; the other had excellent business systems; and then began pursuing the dream of buying a pharmacy of his own.

A few years into the relationship with Ben, Lynne found she was pregnant. They were living in Canberra at the time as Ben had been looking at buying a pharmacy there. Despite some misgivings about their level of commitment to each other, they decided to go ahead with the pregnancy.

'Lynne wasn't sure whether we would stay together but she wanted to have the baby anyway. And because I was adopted, I had a very strong compulsion that if there was a baby coming into the world then I had to be there. So I was determined to make the relationship strong and so was Lynne,' Ben tells me.

Lynne suffered six months of debilitating nausea, something Ben attributes to her feeling apprehensive about whether things would work out between them, combined with her being physically under-resourced for the demands of pregnancy. He says she had spent a decade as a 'bad' vegetarian, the kind of girl who eats the family meal but takes the meat off the plate and so has a very poor intake of protein and iron. Lynne called in sick so many times during the pregnancy that the insurance company she was working for in Canberra was on the point of terminating her employment. As Lynne obviously needed a support network and the pharmacy purchase possibility had faded away, they decided to go back to Sydney, but found the difficulties only intensified.

'We moved back to Sydney, to Thornleigh, an area neither of us had lived in before. The house was dodgy and we were down to one income. Lynne had never managed her finances particularly well and when we went back to Sydney in 1999 she had no work and I found out that she was still paying, at credit card interest rates, her travel bill from 1991. So a lot of my savings to buy a pharmacy went on that. There was no point paying eighteen per cent on a credit card every month. I had a fair bit of resentment about that, I'd say, looking back. And she had resentment too, because she wanted to maintain her independence.'

A baby was added to this tricky mix, one that slept poorly during the day and the night. Lynne found the crying hard to handle. She joined a mother's group but felt she had no-one she could really call on for help. None of her old friends had children yet. Ben left for work at six thirty for a ninety minute commute on public transport and three times a week he didn't get home until nine p.m. He had rugby training after work twice a week and on another night he was involved with Pharmacy Council activities.

By the time Chloe was six months old, Ben and Lynne were fed up with having to squeeze all their family time into the weekends and decided to seek a less pressured lifestyle on the north coast of New South Wales. Ben had been offered a job at a large pharmacy in Forster-Tuncurry as well as the opportunity of eventually buying into the business. With Ben's workplace only five minutes from their new home, Lynne could sleep in while father and daughter enjoyed a couple of hours together each morning.

Towards the end of 2000 they decided to have a second baby, and a third came along in 2003. Lynne continued to be a stay-at-home mum: they had agreed this was best.

'I always wanted to provide for my children the situation where the mother was available for them,' Ben tells me. 'I didn't really want Lynne to work while the kids were growing up. Besides, it didn't matter what job she got, I'd be earning several times the hourly rate that she was.'

I inquire about Lynne's view of the matter.

'She felt the same as I did, until about 2003. Then she really needed to get away from it all but she didn't know what she wanted to do. She was saying, "I'm not happy just looking after the kids and the house – this is not the life I want." One week it would be: "I might think about applying for a job." The next week: "I don't want to do that, I want to study." The following week: "Maybe I'll go and do some charity work." And what happened was that nothing happened. After we left Canberra, she never worked again. And she never did any study either.'

Ben explains that once he was established at the pharmacy in Forster, he rarely spent more than forty hours a week at work. He obviously regards this as verging on part-time for someone in his profession, especially for a younger partner in a very busy practice.

'Lynne could have utilised a couple of days, or one day a week, to do other things, but she never chose to leave the kids. She was incredibly houseproud too. I think she felt it was her job to look after the house and the children. Naturally she got a lot of pleasure out of the kids, but when it wasn't going right it was an extremely heavy burden. But she would not have liked to say that. She really struggled with motherhood. She'd often ask for assurances that she was a good mother, and as a partner trying to be loving, you do that as best you can, but she knew she wasn't the mother that she wanted to be.'

As I listen to this, I notice that I am feeling increasingly sad about how things transpired for Lynne. During the years that Ben was enthusiastically bounding ahead with his professional career, achieving business success, win-ning medals for excellence and flying off to be on govern-ment committees, it sounds like Lynne was sinking into the scenario described by Betty Friedan in *The Feminine Mystique,* losing her sense of self in the role of wife, house-keeper and mother, and becoming increasingly discon-tented with her lot in life.

Apart from intermittently proposing solutions but failing to act on them, and occasionally speculating about separa-tion, Lynne's main way of expressing her unhappiness was through stony silences, a method Ben found quite unnerv-ing.

'There were periods where everything was going along seemingly okay and there were other days that were just dark. I'd come home from work, might get here at ten to six or something, and find Lynne was so cross that she couldn't speak. It was almost like she was peeved that I hadn't been there to help all day. She wasn't one to carry on with a great deal of fanfare; she just wouldn't speak to me. Which was a thousand times worse. I would rather have had a dressing-down. I'm an extroverted person, I like to be involved in an open way, so for someone to close up shop and not talk, and you don't know what they're thinking – you're not carrying a crystal ball – naturally your own mind starts going off in tangents. Lynne knew that it tortured me. So if she was cranky, she just said nothing.'

I ask, 'Didn't Lynne leave the kids with you sometimes so she could have some time for herself?' When I'd been at home with small children, the front door barely had time to close on my arriving husband before I was pushing it open to make my escape, off for a long vigorous walk, to choose new books from the library, or to see a movie with a friend.

Ben's answer leaves me dumbfounded. 'Not really,' he tells me. 'If she did, it would be to go shopping, to do the groceries; not what you'd call a real recharge.'

Lynne's ovarian problems surfaced when she was pregnant with her second child. A benign cyst the size of a grapefruit was aspirated early in 2001, when the foetus was at twelve weeks gestation. The growth returned, so after Nick was born Lynne had an operation to remove the entire ovary. Surprisingly, she conceived again within a year, and Luke arrived in March 2003, on his sister Chloe's fourth birthday. At first, everything was rosy. Ben says that this particular Friday was 'the most magical day you could ever ask for': the birth went smoothly; Chloe and her friends had a great party; Lynne and the baby were home from hospital in time for a family dinner. But as the weekend progressed it became clear Lynne was not at all well. 'By Sunday she still looked fully pregnant. I took her back to hospital and by Wednesday she was so weak that I was holding Luke to her breast so she could feed him.'

The staff at the hospital tried to suggest the distended, flaccid stomach and the extreme fatigue could be symptoms of post-natal depression. Lynne and Ben refused to accept that diagnosis. On Friday afternoon Ben revved himself up for a confrontation, aware that if he didn't act immediately, nothing would happen until the following Monday. Lynne's gynaecologist came in and agreed to operate the next morning.

'He came out from the procedure and informed me they'd pulled out a tumour that was 3.4 litres in size. It was a mucilaginous tumour, a very soft balloon filled with water and when you pushed it, it changed shape. So that meant it hugged around Luke in utero and that was why it was never picked up.'

Ben listened to this, appalled. The gynaecologist had spent the last five days telling them it wasn't a gynaecological problem. Lynne was a longstanding patient of his, but some of her operations had been performed by other doctors because he hadn't been available. Ben knew these doctors had recommended that Lynne receive close monitoring.

'I said to him, "Lynne has a history of ovarian problems. You tell me what Dr. H wrote after her last operation." I pressured him until he eyeballed me and admitted he'd never read the reports. He couldn't even remember that she'd had an ovarian cyst. I was in total disbelief so I was emotionless. If I'd been in any other state I probably would have laid him out on the floor.'

The excised tumour was cut up into one centimetre cubes for analysis. The results indicated that it was borderline malignant and no further treatment was required. This diagnosis was wrong, but the tumour was so large that someone could have spent six months cutting it up without discovering the truth. Seven months later, the gynaecologist sent Lynne to an oncologist because her cancer markers were elevated and she had an umbilical hernia.

'He opened her up and the cancer was all over the remaining ovary, all around the uterus. There were nodules all through the omentum, the fat layer that surrounds the uterus and the organs. It's like a sponge, so you can imagine it would have looked like a cauliflower, when he opened her up.'

Lynne had a full hysterectomy in November 2003 and chemotherapy every three weeks from January through to June. Her parents, who lived in Sydney, came and stayed each time to help her get through the worst of it. A capable, good-natured local woman, Tracy, began working in the house two days a week, doing housekeeping tasks and caring for the children so that Lynne could rest. Ben says that Lynne was very positive throughout these months and all the blood tests were encouraging. They drove down to Newcastle together for the treatments and enjoyed the chance to chat during the two hour trips. On the 1st of July, Lynne went with a girlfriend for the final appointment. 'She felt that everything was sweet, and afterwards they were going to shop and have lunch,' says Ben.

The plans collapsed when the specialist announced that the chemotherapy had only temporarily stunted the cancer; it was now back in a more aggressive way and there was no further treatment available.

The following weeks were dark and desperate. An extreme heaviness descended on Lynne. She was resentful and angry and unhappy. She felt she would not survive without making drastic changes in her life; she spoke again of splitting up. Ben sharply curtailed his days at work, only going in once or twice a week, and organised to sell his share of the pharmacy so that he would be free to devote himself to caring for Lynne and the children.

Lynne's prognosis was six months, but she plummeted so severely, psychologically, emotionally and physically, that Ben thought she might die before the end of July. Her stomach swelled and she began suffering from night sweats so profuse that the liquid dripped from her clothes. One particular night, Ben was roused from sleep seventeen times to see to her or the children, and the next morning he had to get up and go to work. 'There were twelve lots of clothes beside the bed so I must have been up twelve times, because Lynne was too exhausted and too distressed to get the clothes herself. And I got up five times that night to the kids.'

Ben used his private school contacts to arrange appointments to seek opinions from the leading medical specialists in Sydney. One of the radical treatments offered was to open Lynne up, peel the peritoneum off her internal organs, pour chemotherapy drugs into the cavity and let them swill around for an hour before sucking them out and sewing her up again.

'It was real hero medicine, a slim chance of success but if it worked the doctor would come out the hero. He was excited about the opportunity to do this. He said, "You're young, it might make a difference." But we decided against it because the potential for suffering was too great.'

They investigated alternative medicine options – Chinese herbalists, naturopaths, psychics – grasping at any possible hope. They made plans for the coming months, trying to fit in as much as possible. They both knew that the estimate of how much longer Lynne had to live was based on averages and might be wildly inaccurate. 'We had this attitude that it could be three days, three months, three years,' Ben says. 'But the back of our minds were saying – do things now!' They arranged for Lynne's parents to mind the children for a week so that they could attend the next Quest for Life program and booked a family holiday on the Sunshine Coast in Queensland.

In early August, Lynne had a startling resurgence of well-being. She was vibrant and happy, brimming with energy. Ben could hardly believe the turnaround in her mental and physical state. I ask what might have caused the change: was there a shift in her attitude towards hope, or resignation? Ben speculates that having things to look forward to might have helped Lynne to manage her emotions, but notes at the time he'd been treading cautiously and hadn't liked to enquire too closely.

'July was really heavy. It wasn't the sort of thing where you'd say, hey last week was as bad as it could ever be, and this week it's good, let's sit down and talk about it for three hours.'

Ben describes the five days they spent on the Quest for Life program in mid-August as 'the most wonderful bonding moments' they had experienced in a long time. 'We were really close that week. It's the nature of the program and what you learn about. We opened up to communicate about things that we hadn't under our own roof.' They found the meditative techniques taught on the program particularly rewarding. Lynne continued to practice meditation after she returned home.

From the middle of September, Ben watched Lynne growing physically frailer: eating less, spending more time in bed, her threshold for claiming 'a good day' dropping week by week. Ben wanted to be encouraging, he wanted to affirm that she was going well, but he found it heartbreaking to agree that she'd had a good day when he could see her plummeting.

Lynne suffered from diarrhoea, breathlessness, nausea, cramps, pain and night sweats. In the struggle to ease the discomfort and help her sleep, Ben would massage her feet and rearrange her pillows, and fetch teas, heat packs, ice, water, herbs, medication, and dry clothing. Although Lynne was failing physically, she did not sink back into the misery of July. 'I suppose subconsciously she knew the end was in sight, but she wanted to ignore that and keep doing things as best she could. She seemed a lot happier. All her friends would attest to how positive she was and so do I. That's probably in a strange way one of my fonder times. She was so upbeat and inspirational.'

It was during this period that Lynne began preparing a book of memories for her children. One of the entries concerns a particular day in 2001, long before she became ill, when Ben and Chloe had left the house early on a furtive errand:

I was having a sleep-in but unfortunately the phone kept ringing. I finally got up to answer it and found a poem sitting at the top of the stairs inviting me to head to Burgess Beach (our favourite beach). When I arrived I looked down onto the beach where your dad and Chloe had written 'Marry Me' in flowers – too romantic.

Lynne accepted, but the idea went onto the back-burner and the wedding didn't actually take place until a month before she died. They were married at a registry office in Newcastle on the 16th of November 2004; a quiet affair with a couple of close friends and a meal afterwards. Ben took a wheelchair for Lynne but she managed to get through the day without it. In the photos, she is wearing a cream halterneck dress that reveals how gaunt she had become, but she is smiling.

In the final month of her life, Lynne was surrounded by friends and family for much of the time. Her four closest girlfriends came and stayed for a week early in November, then returned at the end of November for two more weeks in response to Lynne telling them that she really was going this time and they needed to come up again to say good-bye. However, the extra people in the house did not lead to any lessening of Ben's workload. If the visitors tried to help with the domestic tasks or the childcare Lynne would say, 'Oh no, you're not here to do that. You're here to spend time with me. Ben can do that.'

'Did you ever feel that you were overworked?' I ask. 'I mean, given the broken sleep on top of everything else?'

'At the time I just would have done anything for her to be peaceful and calm and happy. So, at the time, no. But later, after she died, reflecting on it, I felt that it was unfair that she had driven me so hard. I was probably at the stage where maybe, if I didn't have a strong constitution, that I would have been crook as well. And I thought, geez, that was a senseless thing to do. When we had lots of people here. They could have taken care of the kids and I could have taken Lynne out for a coffee or to sit down and look at the water for half an hour if she wasn't up for a walk. Or I could have done something for myself. I didn't need to be doing breakfast, lunch, dinner, full-time care of the kids, full-time care of her, making sure I settled things if there was an issue with her mum – just trying to be all things, to cover everything.'

I ask my next question very cautiously. 'Would there have been a sense that you were being repaid, for all the times when she thought that you hadn't done enough?'

'Mmm. Maybe. And look, maybe I was carrying a bit of guilt? You know, that the load had been too much for her in the past, and I was trying to make up for it? Later I resented the fact that I didn't have the courage to stand up and say no, this is getting ridiculous. But at the time I just thought: I want her to be happy.'

On one occasion, Lynne's girlfriends took pity on Ben and surreptitiously sent him off for a run along the beach, offering to tell Lynne that he was out fetching milk if she noticed his absence. He remembers the feeling of dry heat on one side of his face and a cold wind from the sea on the other side. He remembers it because the contrast of sensations was repeated several weeks later when he ran on the beach again, on the afternoon of the day that Lynne died.

'I was running along, crying, thinking – why? Why couldn't we have just come down for a walk together? We had so many opportunities and she never wanted to. Why didn't she want to do that? It was ridiculous that we didn't take those chances. Because now I can't ever get them again.'

By December it was clear that Lynne did not have long to live. She struggled, yellowed with jaundice, to Chloe's end of year events at school; she organised presents for an early family Christmas; she spoke of her desire to die at home. She made detailed plans for her own funeral and discussed them calmly and confidently with the person who would conduct the service. She also wrote them down in the book for her children:

I would like Pachelbel's Canon to be played at some point. I would like to be cremated in a white coffin covered in frangipanis. I don't want a religious service but I would like heaven and eternal life to get a mention. I would like my [beloved deceased grandfather] Boppy to be mentioned. I would like 'Songbird' by Christine McVie (Fleetwood Mac) to be played as my coffin disappears. I hope all my family and friends can be here to celebrate my life – so I'd like a big party at our house with lots of wine and yummy food. I would like my ashes to be thrown out to sea one day, hopefully with your dad's. I want to be buried on a Friday so everyone can have a long weekend.

Lynne's friends left on the 10th of December. She had sparked up with all the love and attention and it had seemed that she was not at the point of death after all; but at eight p.m. on the evening of their departure her pain became unbearable and the medication she was on had to be raised to a level that rendered her semi-conscious. 'Friday night was bad; she was drugged out on Saturday; Sunday she could talk but during that night she was really not with us. I was the only one in the room and she called out for her mum that night. And she wasn't the sort of person to say, "Oh Mum, pick me up, give me a hug," as she did that night. So that was pretty intense.'

By Monday morning Ben had been carrying Lynne to the toilet for three days and nights. She was just skin and bone in his arms. He took her into the bathroom for a shower and left her briefly. When he returned, he found she had been incontinent without calling out for him; without even realising.

'I was sort of, not beside myself, but a bit numb to it all. What am I going to do? You know, the three kids are out there, and Lynne's parents, we're all exhausted, we're all emotionally drained and physically done and Lynne's losing it. After I cleaned that up and Lynne went back to bed, the palliative nurse came in and we sat down and I told her what was happening. I still had it in my mind that I had to nurse Lynne to the end at home because that was her wish, but the nurse said, "I think she really needs to go to hospital now." And I said, "Oh, you reckon?" And she said, "It would be a good thing to do now".'

Ben agreed, but says at that point he hadn't fully comprehended that this was the end. The children said goodbye to their mother at the front door. Ben went in the ambulance with Lynne to Manning Base Hospital and stayed overnight. Lynne was given extra morphine and went into a zombie-like state. Ben came home on Tuesday to see the children and to give Lynne's parents and sister a chance to visit.

'They came back about four in the afternoon and her mum and dad said Lynne had been chatting to them. This really did my head in. Because I was thinking, is this me? Is she just not wanting to talk to me – again – all of a sudden? I went back to the hospital, ready to have a conversation with Lynne, which hadn't happened since last Friday, she'd been so out of it. But she was still the same and I realised she couldn't have been chatting with them. It must have just been what they wanted to see, so if she turned over and murmured, they took that as a sign she was responding to their conversation.'

Sitting in a chair beside the unconscious Lynne, Ben distracted himself with his Palm Pilot until about midnight, and then fell asleep on the fold-out bed provided by the hospital. He woke briefly because Lynne groaned, saw that it was only five o'clock, and thought, that's ridiculous,

I'm going back to sleep. Later he realised that was probably her last breath.

Ben says he got through the months after Lynne's death by taking the kids on the road for a while, visiting people: basically running away. 'That routine of getting up and doing the home stuff – by the time January came around, I was thinking, whoah! Right now, I'm not up to doing this shit every day.' They got in the car: they went to Gunnedah, Moree, Sydney, Orange, Sydney again, Queensland. 'We were catching up with close friends and family. We were out having fun. In six weeks I did forty-five hours in the car with the kids. We had one bad hour. So the kids were awesome.'

Ben has been talking to me all afternoon; some of it against the clatter of the children arriving home from preschool and school and interacting animatedly with Tracy, who still comes once a week. Nine year old Chloe, a slight, pale-complexioned strawberry-blonde, has brought out plates of healthy snacks for afternoon tea: rice crackers, olive and hummus dips, carrot and celery sticks. She leans into Ben's side and asks about his day. He puts an arm around her and answers the question with mock seriousness: he was at work until eleven thirty; then he went to Nick's school to help with Maths, as he does every Wednesday; he went back to the pharmacy briefly to cover the lunch period; then finally came home to meet me.

These days Ben works part-time in a pharmacy owned by someone else. He is also establishing himself as a self-employed consultant in diet and nutritional therapy, helping people overcome deficiencies that can cause disease and inhibit well-being. And he's obviously a devoted, hands-on father.

REBECCA

When is the right time to die in the overall course of a lifetime?
The answer is probably: Before or After ... Clearly, before the
all-out attempts to prevent it that leave the dying person with little identity, health or dignity ... The after must apply to norma-
tive ideas of a long life, which is also partly the aim of not letting
people die 'too soon', 'before their time' or before 'everything that
can be done for them is seen to be done for them'.

Allan Kellehear
A Social History of Dying, Cambridge University Press,
2001, p. 236

Genevieve and I went to Brooklet to take care of my
mother when she came home from hospital after a bout
of pneumonia. Chemotherapy had removed her hair, her
immune system and her vigour, and left her thin, bald and
pale.

JANENE CAREY

'I look like Gollum from *Lord of the Rings*,' she said. I felt a pang; I could see the resemblance. But two-year-old Genevieve noticed nothing amiss and was simply entranced by the collection of headgear that Grandma had acquired since we last visited. One afternoon, the three of us spent a hilarious hour sitting in front of the dressing table, laughing at ourselves in the mirror as we modelled all the snugly-fitting cloches, brightly-coloured beanies, soft, floppy elf-hats and haughty-looking turbans.

Some people think small children and gravely ill people should be shielded from each other. My experience has been that little ones are a joyous distraction, a balm for sadness. When Rebecca flew to Ireland to help nurse her father, she took her four-year-old daughter with her. Unlike Genevieve, Emily was old enough to understand what was happening, but she took it in her stride. Grandpa was not well and he might die. That was fine; everything had to die eventually. In the meantime, here he was in his bed in the dining room, watching TV with her, reading stories to her. And being surrounded by love.

I JUST CANNOT

For the first time in ages, I speak to Rebecca Spence at the university gym. Usually we pass each other with a smile and a nod, but as I am only doing stretches and she is sitting on an exercise ball nearby, lifting small hand weights, I decide to unplug my ears from my iPod and mention to her that a mutual friend who left Armidale over a decade ago has just sent me an email announcing the birth of his first child.

As Rebecca and I settle into the first proper conversation that we have had for years, we uncover some surprising parallels in our recent experiences. I am thrilled to hear she has a grant to tell the stories of our local Sudanese immigrants: I had been thinking that their tales of trauma and transplantation should be recorded by somebody. I explain that I am writing stories about home-based palliative care, prompted by the experience of caring for my mother when she was dying of breast cancer. It is Rebecca's turn to look fascinated; she tells me that last year she spent several months in Northern Ireland caring for her father. She says she still isn't sure whether his death was due to his chronic lymphocytic leukemia, or simply his strong disinclination to go on living with it. She describes how she had found herself mediating between Daddy, who could not, or would not, eat; and Mummy, who was angry and bewildered and kept on trying to feed him.

Rebecca is enthusiastic about the idea of participating in my project, so we arrange to meet a few days later to talk about what is involved. I am enthusiastic too: I'm sure she will make an articulate and insightful interviewee. However, I am worried about a couple of things. How can I maintain that I am focusing on Australian families if one of the stories is set in another country? I think about this for some time, before realising that it couldn't be uncommon for those who constitute the overseas-born segment of the Australian population (23.6% in 2007, according to the ABS) to be called 'home' to attend an ailing relative. Therefore, Rebecca's experience could be seen as an authentic Australian story. But why, I wonder, with her academic background, would she want to filter it through me – why not write it herself? When I ask her this question, she answers that she very much wants to tell the story but feels she wouldn't get around to it without the kind of impetus that I will be providing.

There was one other little thing puzzling me, but I was too polite to raise it at that point. So it wasn't until the end of my first interview with Rebecca, when I was quizzing her about names and dates, that I put the question and was told that in Northern Ireland everybody, children and adults alike, refers to their parents as Mummy and Daddy.

Rebecca is in her mid-forties, and has a friendly face with wide-open blue eyes. Although she left Northern Ireland twenty-five years ago, the lilt still lingers in her voice. She was born in Belfast, raised in rural Armagh, and had a Quaker upbringing, more humanist than religious. Her father was the third-generation owner of Spence Bryson, a company that manufactured and sold linen and carpets worldwide; her mother was a fundraiser and organiser for Save the Children, UK. Ralph and Jane married in 1962 and had two daughters; Rebecca, the eldest, and Verity, four years younger.

At eighteen, Rebecca left home to study at Edinburgh University. After finishing her arts degree, she spent three years as a paid volunteer with the Quaker Peace Centre in Cape Town, South Africa, working as a resource officer helping community groups in the black townships to set up facilities for healthcare, education and transport. In 1991, Rebecca came to Australia for a holiday and stayed with a couple of friends from Edinburgh who were living in Sydney. Her plane arrived late at night. The next morning, leaving her friends' Neutral Bay flat and walking down the hill to catch a ferry across the harbour, she was struck by the glorious blue colour of the sky: 'It was like South Africa but there wasn't all that apartheid,' she recalls. What started as a holiday became a permanent relocation. She got a job writing development educational materials for Community Aid Abroad that took her to Armidale. At the local university she did a Masters degree in peace studies and then a PhD on community participation in Northern Ireland's peace-building processes. When I saw her at the gym, she'd recently swapped her academic job for life as a jet-setting consultant, advising organisations in places like Fiji, Papua New Guinea and the Solomon Islands about how to work towards peaceful resolutions to conflict-ridden situations.

With both daughters having flown by 1988 and the family business sold the following year, Ralph and Jane moved to a smaller house in the seaside village of Killough, County Down. Rebecca describes her parents as a very close, typically middle-class couple who shared a lovely life, especially in retirement: they collected Irish (and later, Australian) paintings, they kept a boat in Killough and went sailing, they loved good food, wine and travel, and combined all of these passions by going on foodie holidays to Italy and France with their friends.

'They hardly spent any time apart,' Rebecca tells me. 'They were always doing things together: travelling, sailing, visiting friends. They even did the shopping together. And when they were here in Australia, Daddy would do the dune care work or go bird watching while Mummy was at the beach, but they'd always meet up for lunch.'

'And did they talk to each other a lot?' I ask.

'Oh, they were always talking! They were both extremely interested in current affairs so they talked a lot about that.' Rebecca pauses, then smiles. 'They bickered a lot, as well. They were very good at niggling at each other.'

In 1998, when Ralph was sixty-two years old and Jane was fifty-six, they bought a holiday house at Red Rock, on the north coast of New South Wales, planning to live there for several months of each year. Throughout their first stay, Ralph was unusually lethargic. 'The doctor in Killough had told him he was just taking a while to get over the flu,' recalls Rebecca. 'So we kept giving him tonics and sending him out for walks. Mummy and Daddy went back home and at Easter, Daddy collapsed and was rushed to hospital. His spleen was so enlarged that it was almost bursting. That's when he was diagnosed with CLL.'

Chronic lymphocytic leukemia (CLL) is a slow but progressive disease caused by mutation in a type of white blood cell called lymphocytes. The CLL cells cannot fight infection, as normal lymphocytes do, and over time they begin to crowd out other blood-forming cells in the lymph nodes and bone marrow. Ralph was given chemotherapy pills and made a good recovery. In 2001, he developed a lymphoma in his neck and needed a course of chemotherapy infusions, but apart from this relapse he stayed in good health for most of the decade after his diagnosis. Swapping Irish winters for Australian summers reduced his exposure to colds and flu, and as Jane and Ralph were both sociable and gregarious people, they settled easily into the local community at Red Rock. Ralph became involved in helping to regenerate native vegetation on coastal sand dunes and also studied creative writing and conversational Italian through the University of the Third Age; Jane joined fitness classes and did pottery with the Woolgoolga Arts Centre.

Just before the 2006-2007 summer migration, Jane rang Rebecca and, in a slightly shaky voice, announced: 'Well, he has collected another one.' It was a family joke that Ralph collected cancers. This time it was a skin cancer, a basal cell carcinoma on his right cheek. Rebecca spoke to her father. He thought that given Australia's high rate of skin cancer, it would be best to have his carcinoma removed there. Rebecca and her partner, Peter, made arrangements for Ralph to see a local specialist.

Ralph and Jane flew into Coffs Harbour airport in January, and Rebecca and her four-year-old daughter Emily were waiting to meet them. Rebecca was shocked to see her father looking old and tired. A large bandage on his face concealed a gaping hole where the skin cancer had become ulcerated. The surgery, scheduled for three days later, seemed to go smoothly, with the operation taking place in the morning and Ralph being allowed to go home the same afternoon. The next day he was up early but went back to bed at ten a.m. saying he did not feel well. Later, returning from the beach, Rebecca and her friends found Ralph slumped in a chair.

'He was not sleeping and not unconscious but something in between,' Rebecca tells me. 'He felt very hot. Mummy and I tried to move him to the bed. As we raised him up, Emily shouted, "Look, Grandpa has wet his pants." And indeed he had. My friends said to call an ambulance. Mummy was shaking like a leaf; she turned to me and said, "What are we going to do?"

'I said, "We are not going to panic – that is what we are going to do".'

With that sentence, says Rebecca, the relationship dynamic between herself and her parents shifted. Rebecca, the calm, competent one, took charge.

At the hospital, Ralph seemed confused and disoriented. 'Is he usually this vague?' one of the male nurses asked. Rebecca and her mother exchanged smiles and responded that vague was not a word they would normally use to describe Ralph. Quite the opposite: he was always meticulous, irritatingly precise in every detail. Never vague – not until now.

Cellulitis, an infection in the skin cancer wound, was the initial diagnosis. It failed to respond to treatment and on the tenth day of hospitalisation, golden staph (MRSA) was identified as the culprit. Ralph was moved to an isolation ward and given an intravenous antibiotic drip that cleared the infection within a few days. But he continued to be unwell.

'He came home from hospital in the middle of February 2007, but he just didn't get better,' says Rebecca. 'He was over the MRSA but he kept on getting sick. Bouts of gastro, colds. He had a pain in his jaw as well. He had great difficulty eating. He was always touching his jaw and trying to rub away the pain in it.'

The family debated whether Ralph and Jane should leave at their usual time. 'There was a big talk about whether they should go home in March,' Rebecca tells me. 'And in hindsight, they should have gone home in March. Because he wasn't well enough to stay. But we all kept thinking that he was going to get better. He was just going to get over this cold, or this bout of gastro, or whatever. They went home at the beginning of May, and he was terribly ill. He was terribly frail.'

Dental x-rays taken in Australia had failed to disclose any reason for the pain in the jaw, but when Ralph's haematologist sent him to a maxilla facial surgeon for further investigation, the underlying cause was found to be another lymphoma. Ralph was thrilled by this diagnosis. He'd been suspecting that he had something new, like mouth cancer or throat cancer. Lymphoma was an old foe, one he'd vanquished previously without too much trouble. He said, 'I've had this disease before, I can fight it.'

However, the treatment regime this time around was gruelling: an aggressive form of chemotherapy called CHOP, given once a week for twelve weeks. 'Mummy was stressed beyond all belief,' says Rebecca, 'so I came home in June to take him to the chemo.'

In conjunction with the chemotherapy, Ralph was prescribed a new drug called Rituximab, a monoclonal antibody. While it was being administered intravenously, Ralph's temperature soared and his blood pressure plummeted. Watching this emergency made Rebecca rethink her expectations about how events were going to unfold. 'This was the first day that I thought: my daddy is going to die. It was my first recognition that this was the most likely outcome of the whole scenario.'

Throughout the course of chemotherapy, Ralph had constant diarrhoea and a metallic taste in his mouth that put him off his food. On several occasions, he was too debilitated to tolerate the next dose in his schedule, so the treatment extended until October. By the time it came to an end, he had lost twenty-five kilograms. His appetite never returned. Everybody, including specialists like the haematologist, kept saying that he would get better if only he would eat a bit more and take some exercise. Jane tried to tempt him with the kinds of meals he had always loved: scallops fried in butter and cream sauce, smoked salmon, freshly-caught fish. Soft food, because the lymphoma had cost him several molars. He would manage a few mouthfuls then push the plate away.

Rebecca rang home one day toward the end of November and quickly realised things were falling apart at her parents' place. Her sister, Verity, who had been travelling backwards and forwards between London and Killough, was in the throes of severe morning sickness. Jane and Ralph's beloved ten-year-old dog India had recently, improbably and devastatingly, contracted lymphoma and died. Ralph's bed had been in the dining room for the past few weeks because climbing the stairs of their terrace house had become too taxing; and when Rebecca rang, he'd just gone back into hospital with another fever.

'Should I come over?' offered Rebecca, thinking: I need to be there.

'Oh, no, no, no,' came the response.

'Well then, I'm coming anyway,' she decided.

The relief was palpable. 'Oh, thank God you are.'

The morning after she and Emily arrived, Rebecca got out a few cookery books and said to Ralph, 'Daddy, I know you don't feel like eating anything normal. What do you feel like?'

And he replied, 'You know, I was just lying here thinking of all the lovely things I'd like to eat, if only I could.'

'Why can't you?'

'I don't know. I just cannot.'

At this stage, Ralph could still get out of bed, dress himself with a little bit of help, and walk unaided to a chair where he would sit down and watch television. Rebecca was taking him once a week to the hospital for a check-up, and out for drives in the car so that he could see the ocean. Gradually, even this limited amount of activity became too hard. Ralph didn't have the energy. So they took him to a dietician, who suggested various sustagen-type products. Ralph tried to swallow them but found the taste and texture repugnant. By this time he was down to forty-nine kilograms. I ask Rebecca whether any checks were done to see if the cancer had spread, but she says no: they were waiting for him to get over the chemotherapy before doing more scans, but he never did.

Rebecca wonders whether the bleak prognosis Ralph received from his doctor was a contributing factor. 'The doctor pointed the bone at him. The doctor said, "You know, the lymphoma will come back. This is a progressive disease." Daddy was sitting in a wheelchair and when the doctor said it would come back, I saw his whole body slump. And I thought: he's not able to fight this. He will not survive another dose of chemo.'

In the weeks before Christmas, the hospital bed in the dining room acquired a protective cover for the mattress, a hoist, and a little table on wheels. Ralph was reduced to walking with a Zimmer frame. Even so, he fell over twice. He didn't sustain any injuries, but after each fall, his walking became a little more tentative than before.

'He hated it,' says Rebecca. 'This was not how he wanted his life to be.'

'Did he say that?' I ask. 'Did he say: look at what I've become?'

'He never did. He never once said I'm sick; he never once said I'm dying; he never once said this is shitty. He didn't talk about it, but I think there was a point when he decided that he didn't want to live. Not in this diminished kind of way.'

Throughout December, there was constant conflict over food. Every meal time was a battleground. Rebecca saw that this was the biggest issue that they would have to deal with. Not so much Daddy's illness, his potential dying; but the fact that he and Mummy were going to fight to the bitter end about whether he was going to eat or not.

'Mummy thought that food would make him better, because food was such a basis of their relationship. She was a fabulous cook and they loved going out to restaurants. They'd had all these wonderful experiences of food, and so she couldn't understand that he didn't want it. She kept on trying to force him. And I'd take her aside and say, look, this is not good, you can't force him to eat. It's not going to work.'

Rebecca began trying to get the message across to her family that Ralph might be going to die. 'I kept saying, I don't think he's going to get better. It doesn't seem to me like he's going to get better. We have to prepare for the fact that he's not going to get better. But they wouldn't hear it. They started calling me the prophet of doom.'

Feeling that the household needed something to lift everybody's spirits, Rebecca decided to get a new dog for Christmas. Jane and Emily went with her to the Assisi Animal Sanctuary.

'We were wandering around looking at the dogs trying to work out which one would be best, and we came across this poor little creature. A whippet. He was shivering in the cold and his head was down. I looked at Mummy and Emily and I said, "What do you think?" And Mummy said, "It looks just like your father – all skinny and bony – we'd better get it!"'

Christmas was a big family celebration. Rebecca's uncle and aunt brought all the food and did all the cooking. Ralph acquitted himself well: he sat down at the table and he ate a big piece of turkey, a big piece of smoked salmon, some vegetables, and a generous serve of pudding, consuming all of it with every evidence of enjoyment. 'That was the last meal he ate in his life,' says Rebecca. 'So he had a really good last supper, so to speak.'

She thinks one of the reasons Ralph totally stopped eating was because he found the relentless diarrhoea so unpleasant, especially when he could no longer make it to the toilet in time and had to wear nappies. Rebecca would change the nappies for him and Ralph would apologise for needing her help. 'It's fine,' she'd tell him, 'it's only a couple of years since I was changing nappies so I'm well in the swing of it.'

Ralph went out of the house for the last time on the 31st of December, for a hospital checkup. Later, Rebecca would find herself thinking about what he had seen as they had driven along. 'It was a forty minute drive to the hospital and there's some beautiful scenery on the way. It's lovely countryside. And I wonder, did he know? He might have known that he wouldn't feel like leaving the house again. I wonder what he was taking in as he was looking out. Because he loved nature. Loved birds – he was a really avid bird watcher. And he didn't go out again. He couldn't.'

The district nurses began coming around each week to check Ralph's blood. His haemoglobin was too low and his platelets were very high; on two occasions he was given a home blood transfusion. But still, says Rebecca, the pretence that he might recover was continuing.

'Everyone was still on this silly little game. Even the nurses were saying to him, "If you eat a bit more and exercise a bit more, you'll get stronger." So Mummy was still trying to feed him and he was still refusing. She'd come at him with a glass of sustagen and a straw, but he wouldn't drink it. He'd say: "Take that bloody stuff away from me. I hate that bloody stuff." I told her a couple of times, "We've got to find a way through this. I don't want you to remember your last months with him as fighting".'

'Was she going out and being involved in some of her usual activities?' I ask.

'She was. We were making sure she was going out a lot. But what tended to happen was that she'd sit with her friends and have a couple of bottles of wine. She was drinking way too much. And if she went out on her own, she was so distressed that she'd just wander around the shops. She needed someone with her, to distract her.'

One of the nurses suggested that Ralph could go into respite care for a week, to give everyone a break. The head of social services in the district came to assess the level of care that would be required. He asked Ralph to get out of bed. Rebecca looked at him and said, 'You can't expect him to get out of the bed. He can't. He doesn't do it.'

The next day they received a phone call to say respite care was available, in a neighbouring village. 'It was in a beautiful old castle, a lovely place. But I started thinking: if he leaves the house now he might never come back. He might go into hospital, and I'd rather he was here. So I said to Mummy, I just won't send him. I don't think he's well enough.'

On the 4th of January, Rebecca rang the locum doctor in the village, a woman called Catherine whom Ralph and Jane knew from sailing, and requested a home visit.

'I'd like you to come here because I need to have this difficult conversation with you in front of my mother,' said Rebecca.

'Oh, I can't,' protested the doctor. 'I can't say anything.'

'You must,' Rebecca insisted. 'You don't have to say that he's dying, but you do have to say that this is a likely outcome.'

The doctor came. 'Right, Catherine,' said Rebecca. 'My father hasn't eaten anything for ten days. He hasn't eaten really for six months. What is the likely scenario for someone who doesn't eat?'

'Well, starving yourself to death takes a long time. You'd be surprised how long it takes.'

Jane looked at Rebecca, and then she looked at Catherine. This was the first time a doctor had said the word death.

Rebecca pressed on. 'I feel he's going to die. What do you think, Catherine?'

'Well, I can't say. But when you don't eat and you're this weak, it's a likely outcome.'

Now that the message that Ralph was probably going to die had been delivered by a doctor, it seemed to have an impact. The battles at meal times ceased. Michelle and Christy, the district nurses, became frequent visitors. Christy lived in the village and would pop in several times a day to see how they were going. Rebecca liked both of them, but she became particularly attached to Christy. 'Christy was just fabulous. She had sparkly blue eyes and a bubbly personality and she loved to laugh. Daddy's eyes would twinkle when she came into the room. He loved her and she loved him. She'd say, "Ach, Ralph, that's a terrible mess we're in, isn't it – we'd better change the sheets." And she was great with Mummy too; she'd always give Mummy a hug.'

Ralph caught a chest infection and Rebecca expected that it would turn into pneumonia, the old man's friend, but it didn't. She and Emily were booked to fly home on the 17th of January because Emily was supposed to start kindergarten at the end of the month. Every morning, Rebecca took Harvey, the whippet they'd rescued from the animal shelter, for a short walk along a hawthorn-edged lane up to a vantage point where she could stand and gaze across the water at the Mountains of Mourne – all the while agonising over what she should do. She didn't want to leave, but she didn't want Emily to stay. Although Emily seemed to accept her grandfather's illness quite matter-of-factly, and had plenty of playmates in the village keeping her well entertained, Rebecca felt her daughter had faced enough disruption already and didn't want to add missing the first day of school to the list. Everyone she consulted advised her to go home, except for one of her parents' friends. He told her how much he regretted leaving his dying mother's bedside. Rebecca made a decision: she would stay and Pete would come over from Australia and fly back with Emily.

Word got around that Ralph wasn't eating, and so people started ringing up and asking if they could visit. After overcoming their initial shock at finding him so dreadfully thin, they would sit by the bedside, chatting and reminiscing, sometimes for hours. Ralph, who had little or no pain until the final week, would be quietly responsive and pleased to see them. 'He was such a good patient,' says Rebecca. 'He was lying in the bed, quite calmly. And enjoying the things he could still enjoy. He still read his newspaper every day. He did the sudoku for as long as he could. And he used to have a gin and tonic every night – he wasn't eating but he was still having a gin and tonic.'

Although Ralph did not have cancer pain, prolonged immobility was causing lactic acid to build up in his joints. He became stiff and sore; he started saying 'Ow!' and 'Don't touch me there!' when he was moved as his bedding or clothing was changed. One evening, about ten days before he died, the family noticed that he was whimpering in his sleep. They woke him up and asked what was wrong. Ralph said he was terribly sore. It was eleven thirty p.m. and there were no strong painkillers in the house, because none had been needed before, so Rebecca rang the doctor. He lived in Down Patrick, about six miles away. He sounded reluctant to bestir himself. The family had known this doctor for years and did not have a particularly high opinion of him. Rebecca was furious. 'Get your arse over here now!' she ordered. So he came and gave Ralph his first shot of morphine, which knocked him out cold for twenty-four hours.

Ralph developed a rash on his scrotum and it became painful for him to wear nappies. Michelle brought absorbent blue-backed sheets to go underneath him instead; these could be manoeuvred into place easily and required less frequent changing. Rebecca would go to bed at eleven p.m. and set an alarm for three a.m. so she could get up and check the state of Ralph's sheet. Fortunately, most of his diarrhoea seemed to occur during the day rather than at night. Apart from walking the dog, she was only leaving the house to get basic provisions: more food, more sheets, and more wine for Mummy. She also bought pineapple iced lollies on a stick for Ralph; he didn't like them but they freshened his mouth and kept it moist. As she walked up the main street of the tiny village, she could see people were avoiding the obvious question, so she would casually announce, 'Oh, he's still hanging on.'

Aunt Una came over from Spain to cook for the household, because Rebecca was becoming overtired. One night Rebecca and Una went out for an Indian meal with some friends. When they returned, Ralph's shirt was all wet and Jane was hysterical.

'Verity, what the hell's been going on?' Rebecca asked her sister, who was there for the weekend.

'Well, that's Mummy,' said Verity. 'She's been trying to force-feed him again. And he said, "Get off!" or "Leave me alone!" or something like that, and she thought he said that he never loved her.'

Meanwhile Jane was crying, saying 'He never loved me; he never loved me.'

Rebecca completely lost her temper. 'I was so angry. I said to Mummy, "I have never heard anything so bloody ridiculous in all my life. That man has always been devoted to you! How dare you say this now?"'

Later, when she was calm again, Rebecca was able to recognise this episode as another example of the turmoil and confusion that her mother was suffering. Jane was terrified that she would not be able to cope if Ralph died. She saw his rejection of food as a rejection of her.

Ralph was drinking less and less. A saline drip was brought in to keep him hydrated. Rebecca worried that this was prolonging the dying process. She asked Christy, the nurse, 'Is this drip keeping him alive? Because it's not fair, keeping him alive when he's like this.'

Christy turned the question, saying, 'What do you want to do about the drip?'

Rebecca felt this was a decision she couldn't make. She spoke to her sister and Verity agreed they should get rid of the drip. Convincing the doctors was harder, as having a drip was normal procedure. The district head of palliative care services came to visit the family and discuss the various options relating to hydration and pain relief. Rebecca and Verity made the case that prolonging life at this stage was cruel. 'I'm very interested in how we get through these last days,' said Rebecca, 'because I'm convinced it's the last days we're getting through.'

'Well, we'll bring someone in at night,' said the palliative care services official. 'So that you can get a rest. So that all of you can get a rest.'

The drip was taken away and a very English woman, Julia, who had been a palliative care nurse for twenty-six years, arrived to sit with Ralph at night. She also sat with Jane, who didn't want to go to bed. She took Jane under her wing and talked her through what was going to happen.

I am amazed by this level of support for dying at home. In Australia, you might expect a personal carer to come and wash the patient and change the bed sheets once a day; several times a week you might see a community nurse trained in palliative care; and occasionally the local GP might make a home visit. In Britain, it would seem, you can have a specialist palliative care nurse come to stay with the family overnight; district nurses popping in every few hours throughout the day; hospital nurses visiting to do a home blood transfusion. 'All free,' Rebecca tells me. 'We didn't pay a cent. They call it hospital at home. As far as they were concerned, it saved squillions of pounds.'

As it turned out, the palliative care nurse only came for three nights; Rebecca's assessment of the amount of time left proved correct. Apart from their closest friends, in these last days people stopped visiting, at the family's request. It was snowing and sleeting outside; lovely and warm inside the house. Ralph was on a low-level morphine drip and sleeping more and more. All his favourite music was playing: lots of jazz, lots of classical. Everyone gathered in the kitchen, sitting around talking, and including Ralph in the conversation when he was awake. He would sniff appreciatively as Una concocted her aromatic meals, and she would give him a running commentary on what she was doing.

Although Ralph was now too weak to hold the newspaper and read it himself, he was still interested in hearing the news and enjoyed having someone read the paper to him. One day, Rebecca was reading him a book and she started crying. Ralph responded in an abrupt, fierce tone, 'What's wrong?'

Through her tears, she said, 'Daddy, this is shitty for you. I'm so sad it's ended up like this.'

If she had hoped he might finally talk about his impending death, she was to be disappointed.

'Oh, it's not so bad,' he barked at her. 'Keep reading!'

Another time, it was Jane, fortified by her late-night discussions with Julia, making an attempt to speak candidly:

'It's all right,' she told Ralph. 'You can go now.'

'Where am I going?' asked Ralph, deliberately obtuse.

'I mean, you can go on now. We'll be okay.'

'I've got no intention of going anywhere!'

Rebecca, who had been listening to this exchange with rising incredulity, laughed and said, 'Well, what exactly are your bloody intentions then?' Ralph didn't answer.

The day before Ralph's death, Rebecca felt in need of a break so she went out to have her hair cut. Sitting in the hairdresser's chair, she kept thinking about what she really wanted to say to her father. When she got home, she walked straight into the dining room and said, 'Now look, Daddy, it's all right. I know you're not talking about dying but it's all right. I'm the eldest daughter; I'll look after everybody. I'm the boss of the house now.'

By this point, Ralph was beyond conversation, but he could still communicate. He winked at her.

On the 31st of January, 2008, Christy told them the end

was near. 'His pulse is getting weaker. And he's sleeping more. This is a sign that he's on his way.' Rebecca felt a great relief. She'd spent the previous two weeks thinking, it must be tonight – it can't go on. When the palliative care nurse arrived that afternoon, she agreed that Ralph was going to die fairly soon and suggested that they sit with him.

'So Verity and I held a hand each and we talked him through it,' says Rebecca, reaching for a tissue as she tells me the final part of the story. 'We talked about what a fabulous dad he was, we talked about all the sailing and we told him that he was going on his next journey. It was fantastic. It was the most powerful thing I've ever done. And the pulse got weaker and weaker and he was getting that really laboured breathing – the death rattle. Then it would stop, and we'd ask the nurse, "Is he gone?" Julia would say, "No, not yet, keep talking to him." My mum came in at the last minute and kissed him. We talked him right to the end and through it. We didn't feel him passing – we felt the whole hour of his passing. And it was a sacred, sacred time.'

It was close to ten o'clock at night but Rebecca rang Christy to tell her Ralph had just died and to see if she would come and help her lay him out. Together they washed and dressed his body. When they had finished, two of Ralph's close friends, Dennis and Finbar, asked if they could go in and pray. Rebecca, like the rest of the family, was not religious, but she said no one would mind.

'So they went in and knelt down beside Daddy and they started to say the Hail Mary. And they got through two lines of it and Dennis turned to Finbar and said, "I've forgotten what comes next." And he said, "I don't know either!" So that was the end of that. Daddy would have laughed his head off.'

After the funeral – conducted by the Humanist Society – was over and all of the visitors had dispersed, Rebecca was finally able to satisfy a desire that had remained tantalisingly out of reach whilst she had been a time-pressured carer. On what, in February, should have been a cold, bleak day, she and Harvey left Killough via the lane edged with hawthorn, amid sunshine so bright that it gladdened the heart, and walked southwards mile after mile along the full length of the coastal path, all the way to the beckoning bee-striped tower of St John's Point lighthouse.

MY STORY

I wrote everybody else's stories before making a serious attempt at my own. Of course it existed in embryonic form, as diary entries and fragmented accounts, before the project began, but I put off writing it up fully until I finished the others. As I sat poised to begin, the telephone rang and a teary-voiced Aunty Caroline told me that her brother, my Uncle Jimmy, had just died on the Pacific Highway near his home at Coopernook. A stormy rain-swept afternoon, a tricky turn into fast-moving traffic, a dark-coloured car that he failed to see coming. And, according to Caroline, another significant factor: the date, Friday the 13th of February.

I am not superstitious, but like poor Jimmy I came to feel ambushed by events unfolding from that unpropitious day. It didn't take me long to realise why I'd delayed starting the memoir. The reason was not, as I had assumed, a justifiable sense of complacency about the availability of 'the material'. Instead, it was my reluctance to refresh memories that had mercifully begun to fade. It was dread at the prospect of reviving my awareness of Mum's suffering, and reliving my own turmoil and bewilderment as I tried to care for her adequately. There was no way of avoiding the fact that before I could begin to shape a narrative from the pain and confusion of that time, I had to load it all back into my head.

I tried expressing this to my husband, but his response was: 'Oh, don't do it. You don't have to do it.'

'But what about the people whose stories I've already written?' I said, despairingly. 'They had to dredge through their memories to talk to me. They found the courage to do it. Of course I can't give up now.'

Driving to Uncle Jimmy's funeral, I took the direct route recommended by Google maps, along the Armidale-Kempsey road. The warnings began as soon as the sealed road ended. I'm wary of gravel roads, having skidded on them in the past. Numerous signs clamoured for my attention: Very Narrow Road; Slip Areas; Falling Rocks Do Not Stop; Caution – Logging Trucks Entering. I felt vulnerable sealed in my car, too divorced from the risks outside to be sufficiently vigilant. I turned off the radio and the air-conditioner and wound down the windows. But conditions became steadily worse. I found myself perched on the edge of a mountain, on a ridiculously narrow ribbon of a road, with a vertiginous drop to the green river valley below. For what seemed like forever, I crept along at twenty kilometres an hour, my mouth open in terror. I was a tiny ant negotiating blind corners with no way to turn back and nowhere to stop; my only option to continue on till I reached the end.

Sometimes, you have to wend your way round those hairpin bends of memory even though you can't be sure what incidents will rise to top of mind. You have to traverse those high ledges of emotional fragility and run the risk of sliding over the side. When all is said and done, the views on such a journey are magnificent. And the payback for your persistence, in terms of understanding and acceptance, can be enormous.

KEEPING ON

In May 2006, my father Peter decided his wife's incontinence, vagueness and precarious sense of balance had become too much for him to handle. Anyone who needed this much tending must surely be at death's door. He rang me and said he had just put her into the palliative care unit at St Vincent's Hospital in Lismore.

'You what?' I spluttered. I had doubted his capacity to care for a person with advanced cancer, but I'd never imagined he would surrender the role so abruptly, with no warning. His own health was not an issue: he was superbly fit for a man approaching seventy. The trouble is, I thought, he's been a selfish, bad-tempered bastard all his life and can't become kind, considerate and self-sacrificing just because we need him to.

'Dr Bruce said there'd be a bed for her at the hospital

when it got close to the end,' he told me. 'She's a lot of bother at home, Janene. You've got no idea.'

He was right; I didn't know exactly how she was. I lived in Armidale with my husband Chris, our small business, and our children aged twelve, eleven, eight and four. We were three hundred and fifty kilometres from Brooklet, where my parents lived in the hills behind Byron Bay. When Dad phoned I had been packing my bag to visit for Mother's Day.

It took me years to realise why, whenever I travelled between Armidale and Brooklet, a feeling of anticipation, of being almost there, rose in me as I drove through Grafton, even though I was still a full two hours short of my destination. It came from a sense that this was where my mother's country began. She had left for Sydney at fifteen and not moved back until she was fifty-two years old, but all through my childhood we headed north for our summer holidays, back to the lush green landscapes where her heart still lived, to visit her brothers and sisters, aunts and uncles, in places like Taree, Ulmarra, Clunes and Kyogle.

My mother Pat grew up the eldest of six children, running barefoot and galloping bareback across cattle country hacked from the bush at Toonumbar. Her father regularly drank the wages from his timber-cutting jobs, so the family income was meagre. Their lifestyle resembled one from the late nineteenth more than the mid-twentieth century. The house had no running water or electricity; laundry was boiled in a wood-fired copper; a drum buried in shady ground kept the food cool. At fifteen, with the support of two aunts on her father's side, Pat escaped to Sydney and enrolled as a student nurse at Balmain Hospital.

My parents met when Pat was sixteen and Peter was nineteen. He was her first boyfriend; they met at her first ball. They were married three years later on the 27th of February 1960. The wedding was brought forward so that her mother, who was dying of throat cancer at the age of thirty-nine, could attend. Pat made her own wedding dress as well as a bridesmaid's dress for her sister Caroline, and paid the train fares for her family to come to the wedding.

On her mother's deathbed, Pat promised to watch over the four youngest siblings, whose ages ranged from eight to sixteen. That same week, her father Jim Burke received six thousand pounds compensation for a car accident. Before he could drink it, Pat propelled him around north-western Sydney inspecting houses for sale, so that Caroline, Norman, May and Kathy would have a home near to where she lived at Rydalmere. She was having trouble getting Jim to part with the money until a place they had seen at Asquith went to auction. An inveterate gambler, Jim got caught up in the bidding process and bought the house.

Pat was half an hour away by train from the children at Asquith, but she was a frequent visitor; she sewed their

149

clothes, attended their school functions and recruited the neighbours on either side to keep her informed of any problems. Even so, there were regular crises. Norman skipped school and got in trouble with the police; May began having panic attacks but told no one in the family that she had been gang raped. Pat's new husband and new mother-in-law made it clear that, in their view, her efforts to help the household at Asquith were misplaced and her loyalties misdirected: her job was to look after Peter. Pat remained undeterred; she even managed to persuade Peter to accept guardianship of her youngest sister. Fifteen-year-old Kathy moved in with our family when I was four. My brother Michael was born the following year; both of us grew up regarding our sweet, soft-hearted aunty as more like an older sister.

In 1970 we shifted to Box Hill, a semi-rural, tank-water area on the fringes of Sydney. Over the next twenty-two years, my parents fought the dusty summers and the frosty winters and succeeded in transforming the two acre property into a cornucopia of plant life, much of it edible, all of it decorative. Peter joined the New South Wales Fire Brigade – an occupation that was to send him deaf by the time he was in his early fifties. Pat did night shifts as a first-aid attendant at the Riverstone meatworks but left after three years feeling ground down by lack of sleep and the pressure of constantly having to battle management over lax safety standards. She then picked up the job of teaching sewing to the girls at the local primary school, unaware that the headmaster's wife had relinquished the position because the Department of Education wanted all sewing teachers to become craft teachers. Although she was startled to discover that she would have to teach things like pottery, macramé and copperwork, Pat was deft with her hands and kept ahead of her pupils through evening classes at the high school. She found she relished the creative variety of the job and stayed with it for nine years. In her forties, Pat completed a diploma in welfare studies. She worked as a volunteer for the Smith Family until a paid position became available, helping children from disadvantaged families access the resources and pastoral care they needed to do well at school.

One of the reasons that Mum worked part-time throughout our childhood was that Dad was closefisted with the family finances. In the life story she wrote for her grandchildren, Pat described the conflict that resulted:

When Janene was a little baby and I couldn't earn any money I discovered that Peter considered his income 'his money' and was mean in what he would give me. This made me very angry and upset when I couldn't go out or even buy a birthday gift for my sisters and brothers unless I pleaded for money. This was a side of Peter I had not seen before and I didn't like it one bit. It was as if he was using money to have power and control over me and that created an enormous resentment that lasted for years.

Although I admired my mother's gregarious personality, her hands-on practicality and her willingness to help others, I grew up feeling I was very different from her. She had an active Christian faith and attended church and bible study groups every week, whereas I became a resolute atheist at fourteen. I was always reading, and while Mum was pleased to see me doing well at school, my sedentary habits were alien to her. She rarely sat down with a book during daylight hours: she was always busy, and always exhorting me to be more energetic and useful. But the biggest difference between us was that during my teenage years I began feeling painfully uncomfortable whenever I had to interact with people outside a small trusted circle. My western suburbs high school had few intellectual types and was not particularly well disposed towards them. I shrank into a self-protective shell, only speaking freely to certain teachers and a handful of friends. My social awkwardness and my habit of retreating to my room when visitors came to the house dismayed and embarrassed my mother. She seemed to think if she berated me often enough for being antisocial, she would succeed in changing my behaviour. I suppose she was worried I would grow into a lonely misanthrope, but her warnings and criticisms had the effect of making me feel misunderstood and resentful as well as inadequate. An emotional distance opened between us, and we didn't regain our closeness until I was an adult with children of my own, and had become more tolerant of imperfect parenting.

I left home at eighteen and spent the next decade living in share houses in a variety of suburbs around Sydney University. I finished an arts degree and then worked for IBM for a year while squirreling money away for my first overseas trip. In 1987, when I was twenty-three, I backpacked around Central and South America for eight months. This was an empowering, confidence-boosting experience for me but a source of enormous stress for my mother, due to the somewhat precarious flow of information about how and where I was. During this time, she was also anxiously trying to support her sister May through severe bouts of depression. To Pat's everlasting horror and distress, May committed suicide the following year.

When Peter took an early retirement from the Fire Brigade in 1990 due to industrial deafness, Pat finally achieved her dream of returning to live on the fertile land of the far north coast. They bought a tidy three bedroom brick home five minutes drive from the Federation village of Bangalow, set on twelve green acres sloping from Friday Hut Road to a creek fringed with rainforest. Peter kept himself occupied with a breeding herd of five Murray Grey cows, hand-plucking fireweed from the property, and refining his skills as a fisherman. Pat went in search of new friends: she became a member of the Alstonville Baptist Church, took painting lessons, played tennis regularly and joined an embroidery group. When Peter became resentful about her frequent absences, she started an art group that met in the studio space next to his work shed.

My father's hearing difficulties made him surly and even less inclined to be sociable than he had been previously. When Pat's friends visited, he would alienate them by either dominating the discussion or behaving so rudely that it was obvious their presence was unwelcome. I think he often suspected people were laughing at him, when they were simply amused by conversations that he could not follow.

A cochlear implant in 1998 restored Peter's hearing to a functional level. However, whether fairly or not, Pat thought the stress of living with him while he was deaf caused her breast cancer:

My great fear of cancer became a reality on my mother's birthday, 13th August 1997. I tripped and fell over in the car park in Ballina – whilst examining myself for the possibility of a broken rib I discovered the lump in my breast. Prior to this difficult period there were three years of trying to cope with Peter's rapid slide into total deafness. The misery and frustration created through the inability to communicate effectively with him undermined my health by wrecking

*my nervous system and my immune system. I believe this con-
tributed to my breast cancer and my high blood pressure.*

Pat had a mastectomy, chemotherapy and took the
anti-oestrogen drug Tamoxifen for five years. Just when it
seemed the cancer was beaten, it returned in 2003 on her
chest wall. The doctors told her they would throw everything they had at it: surgery, twelve weeks of chemotherapy, six weeks of radiation therapy. It didn't work. New
tumour sites kept appearing; more treatments were
applied. Her oncologist called it 'spot welding'. A total hip
replacement was performed in April 2004 when the head
of her femur was found to be hollow, eaten away by can-
cerous cells.

Later, it emerged that the chemotherapy Pat had
received was ineffectual against her particularly aggressive
sort of breast cancer. She should have been tested to see if
she needed trastuzumab (more commonly known as Herceptin), a monoclonal antibody that binds to cancer cells
containing high levels of a protein called HER-2. However,
she knew nothing of this until she went to Brisbane for
a second opinion about her treatment options. She never
got a straight answer from her local oncologist as to why
he hadn't checked to see if her cancer was the kind that
responds to Herceptin. Given that every patient receiving
this subsidised drug was costing the health care system
over $50,000 annually, she did wonder whether, as a grey-

haired granny of sixty-three, she had not been considered worth it.

Pat started receiving weekly infusions of Herceptin in September 2004. It kept her free of bone metastases for the next twelve months. Unfortunately, it didn't protect her brain.

On the 8th of June 2005, in the midst of our usual morning rush to get lunches packed and three boys on the school bus, the phone rang. It was my Aunty Caroline, telling me that Mum was in hospital after having some kind of seizure during the night. The cause was still unknown. We speculated about the possibilities: high blood pressure, a stroke, an aneurism? It was perplexing because my mother had seemed, in the last couple of months, to be slightly better. Her recent scans had been clear, she'd reported needing fewer pills for anxiety and had resumed driving as she was suffering less pain in the leg connected to her artificial hip. In fact, during our regular Sunday phone conversation just two days earlier, I had decided she was strong enough for me to risk upsetting her – so I'd finally told her how much I disapproved of what she had done during her last visit to Armidale.

She had come over by herself, on the bus, planning to stay two weeks. Dad, who never liked leaving home for more than a few days, was due to arrive just in time to see me graduate with a Master of Economics degree. I don't

think he'd been informed that the reason for this arrangement was to check how feasible it would be for Mum to
live with us if her health declined, rather than having to
depend on him to look after her. But the trial run was a
dismal failure. Every evening we had some crisis of family
life involving fights, tears, threats and shrieks before bed
time. Chris had gone to an aikido camp in Sydney and, as
I was obviously struggling to maintain some semblance of
order in his absence, Mum presumed her help was needed
in disciplining the children. By the weekend, she was so
outraged by their behaviour that she announced, quite
seriously, that in future she would no longer buy them any
Christmas or birthday gifts. They were spoilt, unhelpful,
argumentative and ungrateful. She would use her money
to fund sanity breaks for me, their frazzled mother,
instead.

I knew her capacity for judging and sentencing well
enough to understand that this was no idle threat. Once,
I would have challenged her immediately, would have said
that the emotional bludgeon she was wielding on three
boisterous boys and a very little girl was far too harsh. But
I knew she had been finding the visit difficult: she was suffering badly from constipation and bloating and no doubt
the discomfort was making her more irritable than usual.
She had been hoping for some quality time with me, but
I had been unable to give her much attention. So, I'd let
the matter rest for a few months. When I finally asked her

about the no-gifts policy, I found her still adamant: taking a stand like this might make the children think about the consequences of their behaviour. But what about the consequences for her relationships with them, I argued? Surely she didn't want to be the bad fairy at every family celebration, her missing gift a constant reminder that she thought her grandchildren were horrible? We left the issue unresolved, both of us distressed by the conversation. So when I heard she'd had a massive seizure two days later, I couldn't help wondering if it was my fault.

It wasn't until I was settling into bed that evening that I remembered a chilling fact about Herceptin. Like many therapeutic drugs, it is unable to cross the blood-brain barrier. A study I had found on the internet, and decided not to mention to my mother, reported one-third of breast cancer patients on Herceptin developed brain tumours.

The next day I had a conference paper to finish, but I knew it would be futile trying to work while my mind was in such turmoil. After leaving my little girl at preschool, I filled in time with errands and a trip to the gym. At midday, I rang Mum at the hospital. The doctor had not been to see her yet but the CT scan of her head had been done. She'd expected an iodine injection, and the uncomfortable process of locating a vein on her hand to take the needle – but they had said they could see clearly enough without the iodine. She hadn't known what that meant, and hadn't liked to ask.

Dad left after a few hours, too impatient to hang around any longer waiting for the results. Fortunately, Aunty Kathy dropped by the hospital after work so she was with Mum when the doctor finally arrived at six thirty to report that multiple brain tumours had been found. The largest, in the right frontal lobe, was about two centimetres across, there was another that was one centimetre wide and there were two dot-sized ones. They were inoperable. Whole brain radiation therapy could be used to shrink them. Temporarily.

After Kathy had finished telling me the awful news, I walked into the kitchen to tell Chris. I cried, and he cried too. Then we got organised. Chris cancelled a business trip to Melbourne the following week, I sent a flurry of emails and arranged for people to look after the dog, the guinea pigs, the mice and the chooks. We left early the next morning for Brooklet.

The next three weeks were a time of heightened emotions. Sadness, which had to be muted because Mum was, as usual, being resolutely positive; and also great deal of anxiety about the impending radiotherapy. But there was a strong sense of mutual support, love, joy and closeness, too. Mum was discharged from St Vincent's within a couple of days, and joined us in a household so full that it felt like Christmas. A constant stream of visitors washed in the front door, bringing food and drinking endless cups of tea. It felt oddly quiet when the tide of people receded, leaving just the four of us, the original family unit. Michael and I had temporarily sloughed off our adult ties, waved our spouses and children goodbye and stayed on in Brooklet: we were going to accompany Mum to Coolangatta for her treatment at John Flynn Hospital.

That hushed afternoon, my brother and I lolled about on our mother's bed as she rested and reminisced, telling us loosely connected tales about her life and the lives of those closest to her. She had always been the lynchpin of the extended family, the one who organised reunions and kept in touch with everybody. I listened intently, and began composing a story called 'Country Cousin', about a fifteen-year-old girl, raw as an uncooked egg, who leaves the bush and comes to Sydney to be a nurse.

When my brother and I sat down to discuss our list of questions with the radiation oncologist, Dr Thomas, we found him quite prepared to be frank. No, radiosurgery was not an option. The only treatment available was palliative, not curative. Whole brain radiation therapy would shrink the tumours, and steroids would reduce the swelling around them. The radiation would damage the brain, but by the time dementia manifested, most patients were succumbing to systemic disease.

'But Mum is on Herceptin,' I said, a surge of hope in my voice. 'So that might stop the cancer spreading in the rest of her body. And how can brain tumours be fatal if they just cause tiredness and swelling – and the swelling can be kept under control with steroids? After all, you can't die of tiredness.'

Grimly, Dr Thomas explained that as the tumours grew bigger inside the fixed cavity of the skull, the brain shifted across the midline and tried to force its way down the spinal column, interfering with the breathing reflex and sending the patient into a coma.

Mum's treatment was delayed for a week because the radiation machines were so heavily booked. Dr Thomas was visibly perturbed when he visited her bedside to relay the information, but Mum chose to misinterpret his embarrassment. She reassured him that she liked the facilities 'at this resort': the spacious ensuite room, the lovely meals, the ocean view from her sixth floor window. It was not hard to distract her from thinking about the real purpose of her stay. There were plenty of visitors, including my cousins, Aunty Caroline's daughters, who came several times, bringing their youngest children with them: a chubby four month old baby boy and a tiny toddling girl. I brought in my half-written Country Cousin story and set Mum to work on filling in the details. Father Russell, a man with an eclectic background who was now ministering to the Anglican flock in Bangalow, arrived one evening to help her meditate. He taught her a mantra: *Om Namo Christaya* – I give myself to Christ. Silently repeating this helped her to bear it when finally, fastened to a metal bed by a claustrophobic metal mask, she began the radiation therapy.

On my last day in Coolangatta, I persuaded Mum to join Dad and myself for an outing. Michael had gone home earlier in the week, and in his absence I'd been exploring the local area. We drove up to the headland at Rainbow-Bay and walked across the grass to a stone bench where Mum could sit with the sun on her back and look at the ocean. I mentioned that the previous night I'd seen a spectacularly expensive new hotel in Dubai on television, a curving silver and blue sheath in the desert by the sea. Mum said her friend Ruth had visited Dubai, and then added, 'She's a lovely person. I wonder if anyone has told her what has happened to me?'

Startled, I spoke without considering the impact of my words. 'But Mum, Ruth came to see you the weekend before we came up here – don't you remember? And Mavis, and Johnny Grice – they all came that weekend.'

She bit her lip, her face suddenly childish with fear. No, she didn't remember the visit by Ruth, or by Mavis. She did remember that Caroline's ex-husband John had come, probably because it was discussed afterwards, as it was unusual.

In the coffee shop later, she talked about being scared of losing her memory. I reassured her that someone who could draw the floor plan of a house that she hadn't seen for fifty years – as she had done, to help me with the story

I was writing – was not losing her memory. I said the memories that made her who she was would not be lost. Laying down new short-term memories was the problem, and that could be due to the medications, the radiation treatment, the tumours or just the stress of everything that was going on. But when she picked up her coffee, her hand shook so badly that she spilt it all over the table and onto the bags we had placed at our feet. Dad made an exasperated noise and stomped away to fetch a cloth. 'I'm afraid of going home, too,' Mum told me, in a small voice. 'I don't want to be left alone in the bedroom with no one to care for me.'

She didn't need to explain: we both knew Dad could be appallingly inconsiderate and bad-tempered exactly when kindness and sympathy were most required. I'd grown up on tales of his selfishness, his callous disregard for other people's needs; in fact, the worst reprimand in my mother's repertoire had always been: *you're just like your father.* As a child, I had accepted her black and white version of events; as an adult, I had come to realise that perhaps I'd missed seeing the shades of grey. Pat was unfailingly generous in the help she gave to others, but she never lost sight of what was owed to her. When she was unwell, or feeling anxious, she could be very demanding, and would insist upon the immediate rectification of trifles – spent flowers in a vase, toilet paper that was too rough – as if willingness to comply was a mark of gratitude and an indication of love.

I responded to her concern about leaving hospital by telling her she was well-loved by many people and there would always be someone to care for her. But inside, I was wondering – who? Who comes to give the sort of care she demands, when a healthy spouse can't, or won't? And even if some saintly person did come, for love or money, for how long would they brave my father's irascibility? Even I habitually limited my visits to three days, all the while monitoring his levels of annoyance, waiting for him to explode over some trivial thing, my stomach knotted with anticipatory outrage.

I spent days on the phone to public and private agencies in the Ballina-Byron district, discovering that although help with housework was not hard to organise, actual caregiving services were woefully under-resourced in the public sector and alarmingly expensive in the private one. Between June and December of 2005 I drove over to Brooklet about once a month, usually with one or both of the youngest children in tow. I saw my mother becoming frailer and older-looking each visit. Her pretty curly hair fell like leaves in autumn, softly carpeting the shoulders of her clothes and forming drifts in the corners of the shower cubicle. She began to shuffle as she walked. She continued to have problems with her short-term memory and would write everything down, in handwriting that grew increasingly tentative and spidery.

Friends and family rallied to provide company and practical assistance. Heather, a spry seventy-nine-year-old from Mum's church in Alstonville, agreed to stock the fridge and freezer with delicious home-cooked food. Aunty Caroline and her husband Bert delayed their big trip around Australia and made short forays instead, returning at regular intervals to park their Winnebago in the orchard. During one such visit, Caroline spent a full day tidying up Mum's neglected garden, and Dad responded by making a snaky remark about clippings left on the grass. I was relieved to hear that Caroline simply laughed.

'I know what Peter's like,' she told me later, on the phone. 'Anything he says is water off a duck's back as far as I'm concerned. I'm here for Patty.'

In March 2006, Mum had a minor seizure while Caroline was driving her to Bangalow. Did this mean the cancer was on the move again? As my mother was proving too vague to be a reliable source of information, I emailed her oncologist directly:

Mum had difficulty understanding/remembering your explanation about why she had the seizure last week, and Dad had difficulty hearing it.

I suggested to my aunts (who asked me to call you) that what you probably said was that the seizure (along with other things we've noticed getting worse over the last few months

*like her balance, urinary incontinence, short-term memory
and general decline in cognitive ability) are all late effects of
the whole brain radiation treatment. Is this right? And is it
classified as 'radiation-induced necrosis' because something
I found on the web suggests that 'hyperbaric oxygen therapy'
can help. Is this an option for Mum? If not, what is her prognosis?*

*The alternative explanation is that the tumours have
started to grow again and are causing pressure/swelling and
other damage. But Mum said that the scans showed no
changes in the size of the tumours.*

Dr Bruce rang me that evening and said it was hard to
know whether what was happening with my mother was
due to the radiation treatment or just disintegration
resulting from the presence of the tumours and the
chronic swelling they cause. He said he had noticed a
marked deterioration in her over the past few months,
both physically and mentally. The shuffle gait was char-
acteristic of frontal lobe syndrome; the cognitive aspects
were basically dementia. He didn't think there was anything medically that could be done to improve her condition. I asked how much longer she had to live. He said two
to three months. Maximum.

I felt leaden with grief and regret. I hadn't seen Mum
since Christmas. I had taken on work as a casual academic
at the University of New England, running tutorials and

marking assignments for a unit in organisational behaviour; had joined a public speaking group, trying to conquer my chronic shyness; and had become a foster carer for the RSPCA, socialising feral-born kittens. I dropped everything and drove to Brooklet the next day.

The house was quiet when I arrived. Mum was sound asleep in bed, curled up looking pale and vulnerable. Dad was outside in the rain feeding molasses to the cows. He came in and made a pot of tea. Mum heard our voices and tottered out of the bedroom, only half-awake. I rushed to her side and kept her on her feet with a hug, then didn't know what to do next. The walker she was supposed to use was nowhere in sight. Finally, I gave her both my hands for balance and went backwards down the hall toward a chair.

I'd brought gifts: a soft t-shirt hand painted with flowers (intended for Mother's Day, but now that seemed too distant); and a picture from Genevieve, depicting a vibrant Grandma with curly multicoloured hair and green splotches. I'd also brought some home-made pizza in case there was nothing for dinner, but Dad had a pre-cooked chicken from Bi-Lo and even prepared the vegetables to go with it. The only contribution required from me was the washing up.

After dinner, Dad settled himself in front of the television as usual, and Mum and I talked. She said she had cried when Dr Bruce told her she would not get better.

She didn't understand why he was trying to frighten her. She wondered if seeing a different oncologist would help – someone who was 'less negative'. My mind whirled with conflicting responses. Dr Bruce was the only oncologist in the district and he always seemed to be rushing. It was quite likely that his patience and his compassion were as constrained as his time. Although I longed for my mother to feel that she was being treated with the utmost kindness and consideration, I saw no point in her switching to another specialist at this stage.

Hesitantly, I suggested that the doctor might be correct in his assessment. Mum clearly did not want to hear this, did not want me to join Dr Bruce in stamping on the tiny flame of hope that she was managing to keep alive. As usual, she invoked the examples of Lance Armstrong, Ian Gawler, Petrea King: the roll call of famous cancer survivors. I wished I had a better instinct for discerning the line between speaking with loving honesty and being too blunt, too cruel. Finally, I said that Dad wouldn't be keen on driving for hours to take her to appointments. It was a diversionary tactic, and it worked: she began relating the latest instance of his thoughtless behaviour. He had used the time she'd been in hospital after her seizure to 'get things done' instead of visiting her. I listened somewhat impatiently, feeling that she wasn't being fair. I had been impressed to see that Dad was taking responsibility for cleaning and meal preparation; in fact, that he was now punctiliously maintaining the domestic order both inside and outside the house. I tried to justify him wanting a break without suggesting that Mum was a burden, but of course she was just that – a grievous, worrying burden. Instead of being pressured to stay constantly by her side, he probably needed some signs of appreciation and opportunities to stand free and recharge.

I went to bed feeling tense and slept poorly. I woke to a morning of looming grey clouds and the conviction that I really needed a good long walk. I didn't want Mum to worry about me if it started raining, so I made a point of telling her that I didn't care about the weather. It's a warm day, I assured her, a bit of rain won't hurt me. No, I didn't want to take a coat; it would make me too hot.

Two kilometres from home, the scattered showers morphed into a torrential downpour. Within ten seconds I was soaked. I walked back through a waterfall of rain, my t-shirt a sodden dripping rag that clung to my body like those provocative opening shots from *Ask the Leyland Brothers*. I capered on the lawn outside my mother's bedroom window and she laughed to see me so drippingly wet. She waved me around to the laundry door and met me there with a big fluffy towel.

Later, standing dried and dressed in Mum's room, I glanced down at the Women's Health Diary she had left lying open on her bedside table. What was written there made me realise not only how shockingly unreliable her short-term memory had become, but also how aware she was of it failing. Alongside the details of her medical appointments, daily symptoms and tablets taken, there was a new kind of entry, a message to herself: *7:30 a.m. – 2 panadol. Janene has gone for a walk in the rain.*

While I was out, Michael had rung to say he was catching the bus from the Sunshine Coast and would be in Byron by two o'clock. We'd wondered if his arrival might scare Mum, but she evinced no surprise at having both her offspring turn up unexpectedly on the same weekend. She was delighted that the four of us could go out for lunch on Sunday. At the Harvest Cafe in Newrybar we shared a bottle of Jacob's Creek Chardonnay with our meals. The wine tasted like liquid gold to me but was too sour for Mum. Michael teased her gently, copying her puckered expressions and proffering sachets of sugar. We had a lovely lunch, marred only by the sorrow of needing a person under each elbow to get Mum in and out of the restaurant.

When I returned to Armidale, Chris, my defacto husband of sixteen years, suggested it was time we got married. I was so taken aback that I quizzed him about his motives. He said he assumed we'd tie the knot eventually and it would be a pity not to have my mother there when we did. Mum, who had always been uneasy about the status of her four illegitimate grandchildren, received the news with joy. I threw myself into wedding planning mode, sought special dispensation to reduce the normal waiting period and chose Yamba as a location that was close enough for my family and not too far for our friends.

Brisk and busy, I had not realised that when I had to stand still for the ceremony, the emotional impact of getting married might catch up with me. I found myself struggling not to cry during the service and was only able to cast little glances at Chris as we said our vows, even though he was regarding me with calm fondness.

In the photographs taken that day, the 22nd of April 2006, Pat is smiling from her wheelchair at the front of every group, flanked by varying combinations of myself and Chris, my brother and his wife, the six grandchildren, her siblings and their children and grandchildren, and Chris's parents from New Zealand. There was nothing she loved more than a big family gathering.

Photographs have always been important in our family as a visual record of the people and events in our lives. Mum and I never left them to languish in drawers: we would take them with us to show people, arrange them tidily in albums stacked in bookcases, display them in frames on walls and shelves. Whenever we visited one another, the arrival routine always included a welcoming cup of tea, a recap of news and a viewing of the latest batch of photographs. Therefore, when my eleven-year-old son Robin and I came to see Mum in the palliative care unit, three weeks after the wedding, what first made me realise how much she had changed was watching her handle the photos.

We drove over on the Friday before Mother's Day. By mid-afternoon we were in Lismore, marching along the twisting corridor linking St Vincent's Private Hospital to the public palliative care unit. The walls were deeply fissured with cracks, as though the two parts of the building were attempting to sever their connection, as though the corridor was an unstable tunnel between the quick and the almost dead. We'd walked this way before, eleven months earlier. Brain metastases are considered a terminal stage of breast cancer, so when Pat had been diagnosed with them back in June, Dr Bruce had transferred her straight to palliative care. This served to put her on their books and to link the family into the support services that would be available *down the track*, a euphemism employed by several of the staff who came to speak to us then.

Having seen her so recently, looking joyous and beautiful at my wedding, I was finding it hard to believe that we had nearly reached the end-point of that track. I felt a mixture of incredulity and anger at my father – I suspected that parking my mother in the palliative care unit had more to do with his convenience than her closeness to death.

When we entered her room we found her sitting in an armchair beside the bed, bright-faced and pleased to see us. 'Oh Mum, what are you doing here?' I sighed, kissing her.

'I don't know,' she replied. 'Your father thought it would be best, but I don't look like I'm dying, do I?'

'No,' I said. 'Let's see if we can have you home for Mother's Day.'

I'd directed the web service that was printing digital photographs of the wedding to post a set to my parents' address. They arrived in Friday's mail, so we took them with us the next day to show them to Mum. She was sitting out of bed in the chair again, but she didn't seem as bright as previously. I handed over a large packet full of photos, sure they would cheer her up, but she shuffled through them clumsily, not looking at any of them closely, almost bending them, almost dropping them. I took the pile from her hands and tried presenting them to her one by one, but she couldn't concentrate, she kept glancing away. The conversation between Dad and Robin seemed to be distracting her, as though too much was going on at once. But when I gave up on the photos and tried to get us all talking together, Mum didn't say much. It was hard work getting answers from her. If she was asked too many questions, she shut her eyes.

When she announced that she needed to go to the toilet – right now – I was alarmed to see how much help she needed. Two people to haul her out of the chair. Someone to steady the walker as she slowly traversed the distance to the ensuite bathroom. Instructions and gentle pushes to turn her around and back her into position so that she could sit on the toilet. Help with taking the nappy off, and putting it back on again. Afterwards, she wanted to get into bed and I saw that this too was an awkward operation. She couldn't swing her legs up without assistance.

I could feel myself choking with tears. I didn't want to see any more. I wanted to escape. I told Mum that I'd promised Robin a treat, a trip to the movies to see *Mission: Impossible III*. We left at ten thirty even though the next session wasn't until one o'clock. I said we'd do some shopping and have lunch. I said I was going to buy an album for the photos so Mum could look at them more easily.

We were gone for five hours. Mum either hadn't understood or didn't remember what we were planning, and had become distressed by our long absence. She'd had the nurse on duty ringing around the family, trying to get my mobile phone number to check that we were all right. I felt like a terrible daughter. My excuses were fine, but I knew they were covering the fact that I'd been running away.

That evening, Kathy rang me at Dad's place and said she'd just visited Pat and thought she seemed more vague and feeble than ever before. 'She couldn't even manage to cut up her own dinner and feed herself,' Kathy told me. 'I tried to talk to her about going home and having an extra carer besides Peter. I said, "We'll do whatever you want,

Patty." But I couldn't get anything out of her. Then a nurse came in to see if she would like some tea and Pat said that she couldn't think because people kept badgering her with questions.'

Later, Caroline rang from Brisbane to find out what was going on. She asked me whether I thought Pat had given up because Peter had put her away to die. I said it was hard to tell. I said I was hoping to bring her home for lunch tomorrow. But when I rang the hospital the next morning, I heard Mum telling the nurse that she wasn't sure about going home. She felt very tired.

At the hospital, Mum didn't seem to know what to do with her Mother's Day gifts, so we opened them for her and handed over the contents: a James Herriot DVD from me, a glowing crystal angel from my father. We sat in her room having lunch together, but it was so painful watching her eat her soup with a wavering arm that I suggested Dad feed it to her. A piece of towelling sitting on the tray proved to be an outsize bib.

Soon after lunch, I stood up and said we should leave and let Mum sleep. She looked at me sadly. 'It seems like I just lasted until the wedding,' she said.

I threw myself across the bed and held her tightly.

'When will you come back?' she asked.

'The school holidays in July,' I said. 'Or before, if you need me.'

'If I need you,' she repeated, her face twisting as if she was going to cry.

While packing to leave Dad's place the next morning, I agonised over my decision to drive straight home without visiting the hospital on the way. I didn't want to go through another emotional leave-taking before getting in the car and driving on the highway. But then I found something Mum had written back in February, a long list of all the distressing symptoms she was experiencing. Problems with her memory, pains in her leg, headaches, dizziness when standing up, concerns about how her handwriting had deteriorated. She would have taken it with her when she went for one of her doctor's appointments. At the bottom of the page, in wobbly writing, it said: *What can be done?*

I drove to the hospital, crying all the way. I walked into the palliative care unit and I wept over my mother. She cried too, but before I left she said, 'You know, I don't feel like I'm going to die today. Or the next day. Or the day after that.'

Tragically, she was right.

JUNE

Caroline and Bert are driving out the gate as I arrive. They reassure me that they aren't leaving yet; they'll be back soon. I greet Michael and Dad, who are playing pool in the flat, then walk quietly through the house to the main bedroom. In the faint light that comes around the edges of the shrouded window I can see my mother sitting up slightly, white-faced, mouth agape, snoring. The hospital bed, with its rails, dominates the room. On the dressing table, previously so neat, stand soothing lotions, talcum powder, bottles promising to relieve indigestion and con-stipation, Lindor chocolate balls, cards, a box of dispos-able latex gloves and a vase of wilting flowers. The cloying scent of deodoriser emanates from the carpeted floor.

How I had dreaded this open-ended visit. You wouldn't want to be anywhere else, someone had told me. Actually, what I really want is to be far away and capable of pretending that none of this is happening.

Her eyes open and she gives me a beautiful smile.

'Hello, Mum,' I say softly.

'Hello, Mum,' she answers.

Aunty Caroline makes it bearable. She has always been a zestful extrovert, someone able to light up dark corners with her crackling wit and exuberance. When she is around it is impossible to be serious and solemn, no matter how dire the situation.

Ten days ago, Caroline brought Pat home from the pal-liative care unit. Michael has been here working alongside her for a week; now I have come so that Caroline can get away for a few days. Before departing, she gives me a crash course in techniques for managing a bedridden patient. How to use the special set of red slippery sheets to roll Pat from one side to another when changing her nappy. How to use the pelican belt to hoist her out of bed and onto the commode, or into the wheelchair. How to tuck small pillows between her legs so her knees and ankles don't chafe together and cause bedsores. How to use humour to dissolve embarrassment into amusement.

I can see that my mother loves the laughter and the silly banter that accompanies Caroline's caregiving. She turns a happy, smiling face toward me, back to her sister, back toward me. I feel like she is trying to tell me: this is how it's done. Don't look so gloomy.

During the days of Caroline's absence, Michael takes charge. He is Nurse 1 and I am Nurse 2, the novice. He puts on a jolly demeanour in front of Mum, but I suspect he is finding the mantle of authority and responsibility stressful. My younger brother is normally the most laid back, easygoing person imaginable; now I find him bossing me about and chivvying me along as though he thinks I might slacken off given the least opportunity. Even the simplest jobs seem to require both of us. When we give Mum her nasty-tasting painkiller, Michael stands on one side of the bed, urging her to have another sip, while I am stationed on the other side, poised to deliver the chaser, a spoonful of icecream.

I'd assumed that Dad would still be playing an active role in the caring, but Michael says it is too hard working with him. He can't hear well enough to cooperate; he's rough and hasty and Mum gets hurt. Apart from feeding Mum her porridge occasionally, the only time he enters her bedroom is to bestow a goodnight kiss. He sleeps in another room now because the hospital bed and the paraphernalia around it take up so much space.

Before I go to bed on my first night, I check if Mum is comfortable. 'I'm frightened,' she tells me. She falls asleep without saying more. The baby monitor is in my room, and I lie awake for hours, waiting for it to summon me, wondering what she meant. Was she trying to tell me that she is afraid of dying? Is she finally ready to talk about that? At three a.m. I am dozing lightly when the monitor begins emitting faint whimpering noises. There is a dirty nappy. I get Michael up to help me change it. As Mum has recently taken a laxative, we haul her out of bed to sit on the commode, but nothing happens. We do the back-to-bed transfer, placing her on her left side this time. She can't turn herself over: we need to vary her position. Before leaving the room, we put on her going-to-sleep music – an ABC Classics collection of Bach pieces called 'Contented Rest'. I drift off as it plays for me, too.

Even more pitiful than Mum's physical dependency is the regression in her ability to communicate. Mostly she parrots back phrases, or begins sentences that falter and remain unfinished: thoughts slipping away before she can marshal the words to express them. Often she cannot give a clear answer to a question requiring more than 'yes' or 'no', but sometimes she surprises us. Like when I finally ask her, 'Why did you say you were frightened last night?'

'I'm frightened of the rails. On the bed,' she tells me.

'They're here to protect you,' I say. 'To stop you falling out. If you forget that you can't get up on your own.'

She looks doubly frightened. Obviously, she had forgotten that.

Caroline returns and Michael goes home to his family. His mother-in-law, who temporarily took over his stay-at-home-dad duties, flies back to Sydney. My parents-in-law from New Zealand are still in Armidale, so I can continue being here with Caroline.

I resume my habit of walking briskly for an hour each morning. Caroline is more sanguine about managing on her own than Michael was. My daily walk is not just exercise, it is a chance to stretch out, an opportunity to think, a stress-reliever. If it's raining when I wake up, I feel cheated. When I damage my achilles tendon, probably by leaning across the bed to lift Mum, it causes me enormous frustration. I still go out for my walks, but often end up hobbling home, my tendon re-inflamed.

Looking after Mum is hard work. Her weight is normal – sixty-four kilograms – but as her brain is no longer communicating properly with the muscles in her body, she feels hefty and awkward when we lift her. Before we move her in and out of bed, or roll her from one position to another, we plan the operation first, then execute it slowly and carefully, to avoid hurting her. In addition to the muscular stiffness and soreness typical of prolonged bed-rest, she has pain in the bones of her groin, hip and spine from the cancer. Community nurses come each morning to give her a bed-bath and fresh pyjamas, but we are responsible for the other twenty-three hours of the day: all the in-and-out of bed manoeuvres, all the wet and dirty nappies, all the changes of clothing and sheets, all the meals and medications, all the middle-of-the night hot-packs and extra panadols that are required.

Sometimes we get it wrong. We mix her medicines with food because she has trouble swallowing them and later discover that our grinding and capsule-emptying activities may have diminished the effectiveness of what we were administering. Occasionally our coordination falters and we almost drop our patient on the floor. After one particularly bungled transfer to the commode, Mum proclaims, 'I think that this system is just not working for me.' We laugh about it afterwards, but it jolts us into taking more care from then on.

Evenings and nights are the hardest times for me. Feeding Mum dinner is one of my least favourite tasks. Breakfast is fine; I open the curtains and the fresh day dances into the room, Mum smiles, the bowl of porridge slips down smoothly. At lunchtime we are often outside, sometimes with a visitor, so the meal takes place in sunshine accompanied by talking and laughter. But the evening meal is a grimly drawn-out process. Mum, tired and cantankerous, chomps each mouthful for an eternity, averting her face if I am too hasty in raising another forkful toward her lips. I get little response to anything I say, but if I stay silent the dimly-lit bedroom fills with the sounds of mastication and I have always hated listening to other people chewing and swallowing. Eventually, I realise that the solution to my martyrdom has been sitting quietly in the corner of the room all along. From then on, dinner is served with a side order of television.

Most nights find me lying awake for hours at a time, unable to sleep. My bed is in a corner of the kitchen/dining room area and the baby monitor is on the nearby dresser, so I am subjected to all the nocturnal noises of the household. Footsteps in the hallway, the flushing of the toilet, the gentle snores and occasional moans from the sickroom. Between two and four in the morning we often have to change a nappy or give Mum extra panadol, and if I wake before I am needed I find I cannot relax back into slumber until the job is done. None of my usual remedies, like reading a book or listening to my iPod, seem to work. What does help is writing extensively in my diary, taking the sad, funny and bewildering events, conversations, thoughts and feelings that are whirling around in my head at the end of each day and lining them up as words on a page so that I can begin to make some sense of them. But such compositions take time. I start to feel desperate about not getting enough sleep.

After just a week of being a full-time carer, I am physically and emotionally exhausted. Miserably, I ask the visiting community nurse: how much longer? She says she can't tell, but she does point out that my mother is still eating and eliminating quite normally – there are no signs of her bodily systems shutting down. I become teary. The nurse thinks I am crying because my mother is going to die, but actually I am crying because I feel sorry for myself. When she finally understands, she suggests that I take a break.

Amazingly, it turns out to be possible. Bonnie, a friend from Pat's schooldays at Toonumbar, agrees to come and help over the long weekend in June. Chris arranges to rent a large house at Red Rock, a coastal town equidistant from Armidale and Brooklet. I spend several days there with my husband, his parents and my children, and then return to Brooklet – not exactly refreshed, but at least feeling capable of continuing.

Caroline and Bonnie tell me that they had to deal with record numbers of copiously dirty nappies while I was away. 'Mudslides in Tassie!' reports Caroline, with a grin.

This is the latest variation on a long-running gag started by Michael. He used to announce 'Snow in Tasmania!' as he sprinkled talcum powder during nappy changes.

I notice that a new card has appeared on the dressing table. Like the others there, it has no words on the front, no 'Get Well Soon' message, just a bright, cheery picture. This one is a butterfly, intricate and dazzlingly beautiful. I pick it up and read the handwriting inside.

'In my Father's house are many rooms ... I am going there to prepare a place for you ... I will take you there to be with me ...' John 14:2-3.

We're praying that God will give you peace and joy as you look forward to seeing Him – He loves you. We do too.

Beside the card is a stamped envelope, so it must have come in the post. I hope that whoever opened it was quick-witted enough to abridge the message before relaying it to my mother. It is signed by a Christian couple who obviously don't understand that Mum is not at all inclined to anticipate the joys of Heaven – not if it means having to die first.

My friend Elizabeth, who lives in Mullumbimby, comes for lunch one day. Mum sits with us out on the patio, cuddled in a fluffy woollen wrap and matching beanie. She's fond of Lizzy. When they met for the first time, twenty years ago, at the front door of my new share house in Redfern, Lizzy welcomed her in with such friendliness and offered so promptly to put the kettle on for a pot of tea, that Mum immediately guessed she was dealing with a country girl. Over lunch, Lizzy nudges the conversation toward the past by asking about the places where Caroline and Pat grew up. Caroline describes galloping home from school, three of them astride the same horse. Then my mother startles us with another one of her rare full sentences: 'What about when Jimmy took off before we were ready and left us sitting in the dirt?'

'Oh, yes!' Caroline flashes laughing blue eyes at her sister. 'It was the last day of school and Patty and I were busy waving goodbye to our friends. Jim thought it was time to go – he didn't notice we weren't holding on – so he gave Bess a kick and she went. Without us!'

'We flew off over her tail,' adds Mum.

'And landed like cartoon characters, sitting like this,' says Caroline, mimicking a person in riding position, 'still facing the same way!'

Not all of our visitors are so successful at drawing Mum into conversation. Joyce comes one rainy afternoon, a short, slight, elderly lady with permed grey hair. She hands me a plastic container sparsely filled with chocolate macadamia slice and suggests that I freshen it up in the microwave. Although she looks at my mother as she speaks, the content sounds as if it is meant for me. 'Pat, you were one of the first friends I made when we moved here from Sydney after Bob retired. Six years ago. We were in the same bible study group, weren't we?'

Mum sips the tea that I hold to her lips, obediently breaks pieces of the stale slice with her teeth and eats them, but says nothing.

'What were you doing before you retired up here?' I ask Joyce, hoping she might regale us with some interesting stories. Caroline is checking emails in her room, so she can't help me. But Joyce delivers a dead-end response, with a tinge of rebuke.

'Oh, a mother never retires. You know that, don't you, Pat?'

Mum nods, slightly. It occurs to me that given the variety of jobs and interests she's had throughout her life, she would never have needed to respond defensively to such a question. If called upon to describe what she did, she could always say more than *mother*.

I decide to drop another question into the void. I don't know much about Joyce, but I do know where she lives. 'I haven't been to Alstonville,' I tell her, nudging the plate of chocolate macadamia slice in her direction. 'What's it like? How big a town is it?'

Joyce waves her hand, dismissing the slice and the question too. 'Oh, I don't know. What would you say the population of Alstonville is, Pat?'

I am struck dumb. Does this woman really expect my mother to recall facts and figures?

Joyce eventually fills the silence with chatter about her family. I sketch a profile of myself, but find she already knows a fair bit about me. It seems that Mum kept all her friends well briefed on what my brother and I were up to.

Mum and Dad's ancient Labrador flops down on the patio outside the glass door. Joyce glances at him. 'What's your dog's name, Pat?' she asks.

I hold my breath. Mum looks at Joyce, her mouth slightly open. We all wait for an answer that doesn't come.

'Monty,' I blurt.

Suddenly I am angry. What is this – some kind of test? I picture Joyce at church the next Sunday, reporting the pitiful decline in Pat's cognitive capacity to a fascinated circle of acquaintances. I stand up. 'I think Mum's tired,' I announce. 'I need to put her back to bed now.'

Later that afternoon, another friend from the Alstonville congregation arrives. It is Heather, carrying a cardboard box full of home-cooked meals for us: pumpkin soup, lamb casserole, chicken curry, several meat pies, even a sticky date pudding with butterscotch sauce. As we transfer the food to plastic containers and stack it in the fridge and freezer, we talk about encouraging more friends to visit. Many have been staying away because they think Pat is not up to having conversations. 'She likes being a listener,' I explain. 'She finds it hard to think when people ask her something directly. It's best if they just chat, and she'll join in if she can.'

'Of course,' replies Heather, quite matter-of-factly. 'No one with any sense would ask her lots of questions.'

Caroline's daughter, Rebecca, rings to say that Bert is missing her and fretting about their aborted travel plans and his own advancing age. Caroline is not feeling the best herself: she's been having pain in her neck and upper arm and can barely reach up to brush her hair. I give her a back massage but don't touch the sore arm. She said she felt something go twang in there and it was probably one of her frayed tendons. A lifetime spent cleaning houses and shopping centres has left her with chronic rotator cuff injuries. She doesn't often mention the pain and when she does, she makes light of it. She says that one day her arms will drop off completely and she'll be cured.

I urge her to take a break when I go home. We can put Mum back into the palliative care unit for a little while, I say. For respite care. Caroline eventually agrees but looks guilt-ridden. She starts concocting a plausible story to explain her defection. 'I'll tell Pat the solicitors in Brisbane want to see me about the court case,' she tells me, referring to a pending class action against a South Australian nut farm in which she has shares. 'And Bert is driving down to pick me up.'

I wish she would skip the subterfuge and all the associated anxiety about whether her sister will see through it, and just say – Pat, you'll be well cared for in there and I need a rest. I'll come back in two weeks and take you home.

A few days before I am due to leave, Dad invites the pastor from the church at Alstonville to come and talk to us about a memorial service. Caroline and I feel uncomfortable about the timing of this, but for some reason my father seems to think it is important to have everything well organised in advance.

It is a bright sunny day when Pastor John arrives. He asks to say hello to Pat, so we take him in to see her. She is sitting up in bed, freshly washed, looking alert. Caroline and I get morning tea ready and put it on the patio. I think Mum is expecting to be brought out to join the party but given what they plan to talk about, we have decided to leave her in bed.

I spend a few minutes listening to Dad present his reasons for preferring cremation over burial, then go back inside to deliver a piece of custard tart and a drink to my mother. 'I've got your morning tea,' I say brightly as I enter the bedroom. She gives me a sharp look, and I wonder what she is thinking.

My father is not a churchgoing man, but he spends more than an hour unburdening himself to Pastor John, relating the stages of my mother's mental and physical deterioration. It makes me realise that we probably haven't been giving him enough opportunities to talk about his feelings. 'There's one day I'll never forget,' he tells the minister. 'She was still able to get around using the walker, with a bit of help, and she decided she wanted to put new elastic in some underwear. So I took her over to the flat and left her there for about twenty minutes. When I came back I found her sitting in front of the sewing machine, crying.' Dad pauses to blow his nose vigorously. 'She couldn't remember how to use it. It broke my heart. Seeing her crying because she was unable to do this simple task that she'd set herself.'

Before Pastor John leaves, my father takes him back to the bedroom to speak to Mum again. While they are in there, I walk past the baby monitor and hear Dad spilling the beans about the respite care arrangements. Caroline's latest idea had been not to tell Pat about going back to hospital until closer to the date, and to get the nurse to put it forward as a way of allowing the doctors to assess her condition.

I find Caroline around the side of the house, hanging out the washing. She is appalled when I relay my news, but to my surprise behaves as cheerily as ever in our subsequent dealings with Mum.

That night, I leave the television off as I am feeding my mother her dinner. 'You know I'm going home this weekend,' I venture. 'Bonnie's coming over for a few days to help Caroline.'

My remark hangs in the air. Mum continues eating, slowly and sombrely.

Several hours after I arrive home, Caroline rings. She says Pat has just had a seizure that lasted for ten minutes. She has called an ambulance.

It is a Sunday and as there is no doctor available to admit her to St Vincent's, Pat is taken to Lismore Base Hospital. Two nurses are on duty in the ward: one is scurrying around doing everything; the other is attending to paperwork. Kathy, Bonnie and Caroline end up staying at the hospital for the next six hours, until Pat is settled for the night, unwilling to leave because the care on offer seems so inadequate. They request a meal for Pat, and when it finally comes, they cut it up and feed it to her; they wait an hour to receive a basin of water, so they can change her dirty nappy; they administer the medications she needs at six and at ten o'clock.

The next day, Caroline makes sure Pat is transferred to the palliative care unit at St Vincent's. She gives them a copy of the document I had prepared before I left, containing information about my mother's capabilities and her medications, and the caregiving routines we have been following at home. The staff at Lismore Base had barely glanced at it; St Vincent's take note of my comment that Pat is unlikely to use a buzzer and put her in a room facing the nurses' desk so that they can keep an eye on her.

The palliative care unit at St Vincent's has only nine beds and a policy of sharing them around. Long stays are discouraged: the beds are for treating and stabilising symptoms, temporary respite care and end-of-life care. After Mum has been there for a week, the unit manager organises a family planning meeting to discuss future arrangements for her care. Caroline and Michael send their apologies, Dad and Kathy attend in person, and I participate via speaker phone. Prior to the meeting, Dr Bruce conveys his view that Pat Carey is deteriorating more slowly than he had anticipated and requires nursing care but not hospital care at this stage.

I explain that although Caroline is willing to take Mum home in two weeks time, she can't manage the caregiving by herself without risking her own physical wellbeing. Neither my brother nor I are available for extended periods because both of us look after our children while our spouses work. I say that my father is not a good helper because of his hearing problems and his impatience.

One of the staff members suggests that the family investigate local nursing homes. This limbo land of institutionalised care is the outcome we have all been struggling so hard to avoid. My mother's views on the subject have always been quite clear. 'If you put me in a home when I'm old, I'll never forgive you,' she used to tell us.

Dad clears his throat. He says gruffly that he saw some dreadful sights in nursing homes when he was a fireman.

They assure us that the standards are more rigorously policed these days. I mention the long waiting lists. They reiterate that it is worth applying for a place. They tell us that if Pat cannot be managed at home, they will keep her until a nursing home can take her.

JULY

As my eldest son Tim and I drive into Lismore, the lady from Mulhaven rings me. She hasn't been able to get hold of my father to tell him that our appointment to view the nursing home has been moved forward by half an hour. I ring the palliative care unit to see if Dad is there visiting Mum. He is, so I ask them to pass on the message.

The person responsible for our tour of the facilities takes us into a four-bed ward. It is profoundly depressing. Each person has a tiny bit of space demarcated by curtain railings. They lie cocooned in their beds like ancient shrivelled husks. Our guide points out the advantages of a shared ward – company, more visitors, more attention from the nurses – but all I can see is the last sad stage of life on very public display.

Tim and I go to St Vincent's and find Mum watching television. 'Where's Peter?' she asks, sounding angry.

'He's gone home,' I say. 'He came to see you this afternoon. Before he met us at the nursing home. He said you were asleep some of the time but you woke up while he was here.'

She laughs in a scornful way. Clearly she doesn't believe me. I try talking to her about going into a nursing home. I say that we hadn't liked the look of Mulhaven Lismore but the new Mulhaven at Alstonville was supposed to be a lot nicer. I ask if she would want to be in a shared room, for the company, or to have a room of her own? She says, quite coherently, that it would depend on the cost. I explain that the cost is the same, it is more about availability.

Encouraged by this one answer, I ask her too many questions. She stops responding. I walk over to read the cards on top of her small refrigerator. One is a letter from her friend Diana describing how she is managing after her husband's death. I am absorbed in reading it when Tim calls out sharply to me. My mother is still conscious, but her arms, legs and face are twitching and contorting. I yell, 'Nurse! Mum's having a seizure!'

A nurse comes immediately with drops to place under my mother's tongue. I take Tim out of the room. His customary adolescent bravado has deserted him; he looks upset and scared. I give him a big hug.

Mum is panting and dazed, so we leave. On the drive to Dad's place, Tim asks, 'Did I make her have the seizure? She was looking right at me when she started.'

'Of course not, sweetheart,' I say. 'They just happen sometimes. You didn't cause it.'

But I wonder if it was me, with all my talk of nursing homes.

My sons Tim and Robin were born seventeen months apart and have always regarded each other with implacable rivalry. Therefore, the one full day in Lismore with Tim has a predetermined format: like Robin's visit two months earlier, there must be sushi for lunch and a trip to the cinema.

We walk into Mum's room in the morning just as the nurses are preparing to lift her out of bed and deposit her into a reclining armchair. I watch with interest as they fasten the pelican belt around her middle and then slide it up the ribcage in order to avoid trapping her breasts. We always used to bind her up like an Amazon warrior. This method looks much more comfortable.

Morning tea arrives and I help Mum to drink her tea and eat a slice of pink-iced buttered bun. Today, I am determinedly chatty. I recount the story behind Chris's recent trip to Casualty to have some excruciatingly painful stitches put in his thumbnail. Driving to town for a business meeting, we had met a fat corgi wandering down the middle of the road in a hundred kilometre per hour zone. We stopped to see if it belonged in a nearby property. As we approached it rolled over on its back submissively, but when Chris took hold of its collar, it growled. He muzzled it with his other hand and asked me to read the tag on its collar. I was gingerly doing so when the corgi got its jaw free and macerated Chris's thumb. Various people subsequently informed us that aged corgis are renowned for being bad-tempered and vicious. 'Chris says next time he sees a dog on the road, he's not going to swerve, let alone stop,' I conclude. Mum looks at me blankly. I feel like I am blathering.

Tim and I go to see *Superman Returns*. I hope it will be like the first one – a strong story tinged with ironic humour – but it takes itself very seriously and has disturbing scenes of people being thrown around in an aeroplane crash, people almost drowning as a boat sinks, and Superman being savagely beaten after having slivers of kryptonite inserted into his back. Just like when I saw *Mission Impossible* with Robin, I find myself watching an action-packed, nerve-jangling fiction that fails to provide any escape from the dreadfulness of the real world.

As we walk back down the long corridors to palliative care, my mobile rings. It's Caroline. Given the prohibition on using mobile phones in the hospital, I tell her she will have to stay in my bag until I get to Mum's room. She is amused by that. I let her out on the balcony and tell her about yesterday's seizure and today's revelation regarding the pelican belt. Mum is still sitting in the armchair, tired and uncommunicative. She has been in the same position for over four hours. I make sure she is put back into bed before we leave.

The next day, Tim and I stop at the hospital on our way home and to our delight we find Mum is listening and responding to us remarkably well, better than she has at any time since the wedding. She even feeds herself when the morning tea arrives. It is a Sao biscuit with a cheese slice on top, and as I am holding it to her mouth, she reaches up and curls her fingers around it. I think – why not? She hasn't had her bed-bath yet so the mess won't matter. She proceeds to eat it all by herself, dropping only one small piece. I resist handing over the tea until half of it is safely gone, then I let her have the cup and she drinks the rest.

I allow a tiny tendril of hope to unfurl in my mind. Maybe, if the deterioration was a side-effect of the treatment, she might be through the worst of it and now her brain might be starting to recover? I drive back to Armidale feeling unusually happy. Even if today was an aberration – which I know is the most likely explanation – it was lovely to have witnessed it.

On the 17th of July, I email my brother:

Hi Michael,
When I spoke to Caroline this evening, she was expecting
the ambulance with Mum to arrive soon. She doesn't have

a helper as Bert is not keen and Mavis and Bonnie both have flu, but it sounds like tools and techniques have been upgraded so things should be okay. They've finally got a hoist. She and Kathy both had a turn as patient to see how to fit the sling. Also Carol says she's going to leave the slippery sheets on the bed permanently, under the draw sheet (like they were doing in hospital) so there is no need to shove them in and out all the time. Apparently you just pull on the draw sheet and the top red one and they slide against the bottom red one. Dad agreed to cut down a couple of trees near the gate to get the bus in. Bert and Caroline are staying in the house, but having the Winnebago there means they can go off for short breaks.

Love,

Janene

A week later, I ring Caroline and find her having a difficult day. She mentions that she has hurt her arm again and can't even use it to drink a cup of coffee. Bert and Dad went out fishing early in the morning and so no one was there to help her change the bed when Mum produced a dirty nappy that overflowed onto the sheets.

I commiserate with her and then ask, 'Did Dad look at the information on nursing home charges that I emailed him?'

'Yeesss,' says Caroline, drawing out the syllable in a way that suggests the news is not good. 'He said it was going to cost him five hundred a week and he couldn't afford that so he might as well forget about applying. I got a bit snappy with him. I said: "Well, what *are* you going to do, Peter?"'

My father decides that what he is going to do is seek power of attorney over his wife's financial affairs. For tax reasons he has placed most of their investment money in her name. He will need to withdraw some of it for the nursing home fees, but Pat is no longer able to sign her name legibly.

Kathy arranges for a solicitor from her workplace to come and witness Pat making a mark to indicate that she agrees to the power of attorney arrangement. The day after the solicitor's visit to Brooklet, Kathy rings me with a full account of what happened. The argument that Peter needed access to the investments in order to pay for her care was put repeatedly, but Pat failed to say or do anything that could be interpreted as consent. Possibly she was not lucid enough to comprehend the request; possibly she understood all too well and was deliberately holding out. Ceding total financial control to my father may have seemed a risky, retrograde step, given how she had battled him throughout their married life for access to discretionary funds. Alternatively, she may have been taking a stand against being sent to a nursing home. The solicitor, an enormously overweight walrus of a man who had come straight from work, sat by the bedside until nine p.m. explaining, instructing and cajoling.

'I roused on Pat after he left,' Kathy tells me. 'I said, "You made poor Terence sit here for three hours. He missed his dinner because of you!" And guess what? Quick as a flash, she said: "So? Didn't look like he needed it!"'

I can't help laughing. I treasure this kind of riposte: it proves that there is still someone recognisable as my mother inside the oversized infant she has become. However, what Kathy says next is not funny at all.

'Apparently your Dad's like a bear with a sore head at the moment. Caroline says he's been clanging and banging around the place and muttering that it's his money. This morning he was outside doing some pruning, and when Bert went to see if he wanted a hand, Peter gave him such a shove that he almost knocked him to the ground.'

The poisonous atmosphere my father generates is so pervasive that by the end of the day even the sisters are at loggerheads. 'It took me till ten o'clock to finish giving your mum her dinner,' Caroline tells me. 'She was eating so slowly. I think something was hurting somewhere. I tried everything I could think of to make her more comfortable but nothing was working and she wouldn't answer any of my questions. Then I asked if she wanted a drink of water and she shouted at me, "For God's sake, Caroline!" and I yelled right back, "For God's sake, Pat!

I'm not a trained nurse but I'm doing my best! I hate to see you in pain but you won't tell me how I can help!"'

AUGUST

Suddenly, everything speeds up. Dad applies to the Guardianship Tribunal for a financial management order, sorts out some errors in the Centrelink assessment, finds a nursing home with a vacancy and tells us that he's arranged for Pat to move in on Monday.

I feel deeply ambivalent about this. I realise the current arrangements are fast becoming untenable, but we know nothing about the place that Dad has selected. We had been hoping Mum would get into the Mulhaven at Alstonville, because it is linked to her own Baptist Church and she has friends who visit there regularly. I ring and ask Dad to take his paperwork to Mulhaven, even though we have been told that it has a long waiting list. He does so, and a miracle occurs, or perhaps some of Mum's church friends have been pulling strings on her behalf. They have a high care bed, available immediately.

I drive over and tour the facilities with Kathy. Everything is spacious, clean and attractive-looking. Mum will have an ensuite room overlooking a ferny courtyard containing a bird bath. We meet a nurse-manager with a warm, sympathetic manner who suggests we bring some of Pat's things over before she arrives, to make the room look more welcoming. I ask if we are allowed to hang paintings on the wall, and she says yes.

Caroline is hoping we can pretend that the move is temporary, that it is just for respite care. I don't want to do this. 'She'll know it's not true,' I say. 'And you've got absolutely nothing to feel guilty about. You've been the most fantastic, loving, caring sister anyone could ever have.'

I don't know how appropriate it is to broach the issue of going into a nursing home while feeding someone breakfast, but I do it anyway. I give Mum a full description of Mulhaven in Alstonville and stress how remarkable it is that they have a place available. I don't mention that she is moving in on Monday. Mum displays a flicker of interest and then her face closes down again.

Kathy arrives mid-morning and she talks up Mulhaven with great enthusiasm. Slowly and carefully, Mum says, 'I think I am looking forward to going to Mulhaven.'

But it is unclear to me whether she is expressing happiness or doubt.

On the day of her departure, Mum falls asleep after eating her porridge and I creep into her room to spirit away her audio player, her tapes and CDs, the Petrea King rainbow-coloured ribbon from the bedhead and the box of lotions and creams from the dressing table. Furtively, I disassemble her life in that room as she sleeps. Before leaving, I stand for a moment in her walk-in wardrobe, looking at all the clothes that we are not taking. As it is so difficult to thread her body into clothing, she wears mostly soft, stretchy items that have been opened in the back and made to fasten with Velcro.

People have been telling us that we must be feeling 'relieved', 'glad' and even 'happy' to have found a nursing home place for Pat. Actually, my predominant response is anxiety. She is so dependent and helpless. With all my heart I wish she could be her old demanding self again, capable of insisting that her wants and needs receive the attention they deserve. Being unable to communicate leaves her extremely vulnerable now that she is going into an institution to be cared for by strangers. As we have seen, her only form of protest is to withhold cooperation: not answer questions, not swallow tablets, not chew her food up quickly enough, not open her mouth for the next spoonful. It is a very tenuous form of power. Just a bluff, really. An indifferent carer could easily just walk away.

It occurs to me the word 'kindness' probably has its roots in 'kin', family, the circle of people who love you. I fervently hope that the strangers who are to be my mother's caregivers from now on will be kind, in the fullest, most warm-hearted sense of the word.

The following weekend, I ring Mulhaven and speak to a cheerful male nurse called Alan. When I ask him if Mum seems happy about being there, he sounds surprised that there could be any doubt. He tells me that my mother is 'a lovely lady to care for', that she had a spa bath scented with lavender oil this morning, and that she and my aunts have gone to the church service being held in the recreation hall.

'I spent most of the service crying,' says Kathy, when she phones me that evening. 'The pastor said afterwards, "I didn't think my service was that upsetting!" But I was just so happy to see Pat enjoying herself. Her face lit up when we wheeled her in and she saw people she knew. And she was even singing along to the hymns!'

I write Mum the first of a series of chatty letters that I will post to Mulhaven over the next few months. A friend suggested this; she also has a parent in a distant nursing home who is discouragingly silent on the telephone. I write that the boys are playing outside with a big cardboard box and a large water pistol, that Genevieve is on antibiotics for a sore ear, and that I have been going for bushwalks with the Armidale Athletics Club. I mention that I heard she enjoyed the church service and promise that we will be over to see her soon. I keep the tone light and breezy despite the desolation I am feeling. I miss the lively, loving interactions we used to have on the phone every Sunday. I miss the to and fro of thoughtful conversation, the exchange of important and trivial information about each other's lives. I miss the sound of her warm, intelligent voice in my ear. I miss my mother profoundly, and she is not even dead yet.

SEPTEMBER/OCTOBER

My father drives the twenty kilometres between Brooklet and Alstonville to visit his wife every second day. He stays at the nursing home for about an hour and feeds her lunch if it arrives while he is there.

I know Mum had feared that he might stop coming to see her. A few days after she moved into Mulhaven, she startled everyone in her room by calling out loudly, resonantly, just as he was leaving: 'Don't you forget me!'

I visit once in September, briefly, on my way back from Brisbane. In October, during the school holidays, I take the whole family and we rent a beachside cabin at nearby Evans Head.

When we troop into Mum's room at Mulhaven, she smiles at us and nods in response to our greetings. She doesn't look like she is sitting comfortably – she is on a slant – so Chris and I straighten her up. The children are pleased to see a large framed photograph of themselves on prominent display. They roam around, fingering the lucky bamboo plants and exclaiming over the pictures of Michael and myself as three-year-olds. Genevieve picks up the crystal angel that my father gave to Mum. It is obviously a treasured possession, with pride of place on the crowded bedside cabinet. I take it from her hands and turn it on, and it glows gently.

Care assistants ask us to wait outside for ten minutes so they can give Mum a wash and get her dressed. Chris decides to take the kids to Ballina to buy provisions and I wander around the grounds of the nursing home. I go into the Social Centre, where they hold the church services. I see they have a piano; it occurs to me that tomorrow we could bring Mum over to hear Robin and Linden play. A friendly lady emerges from a side room and gives me a guided tour. She even insists on taking me into the training room and explaining its many beneficial features. Later, Chris also goes for a wander, encounters the same lady, receives the same treatment, and is similarly bemused.

I find Mum parked in the dining room. Her lunch arrives and I feed it to her: mushy meat and gravy with mushy potato and mushy peas, followed by icecream and jelly. One of the staff approaches and tells me there is a problem with the split backs. For a moment I have no idea what she means, then I realise she is referring to my mother's clothing. Apparently Mum almost ran out of clothes over the long weekend. I go back to her room and do an inventory of the wardrobe. I find a dozen items that have been split up the back and lay them out in piles on the bed – summer and winter, sleepwear and normal clothes. I ask the nurses to tell me what is lacking and

they say every item is inadequate. Caroline hadn't wanted
to cut them all the way up as she thought Pat's shoulders
would be cold, but the nurses say each one must be totally
sundered and have one small fastening at the neck. They
tell me Evan's Head has a good second-hand clothes shop,
so I go there afterwards and buy two generous-sized summer dresses with a dropped waist, one floral top and two
large t-shirt style nighties, all in soft, stretchy cotton. I also
arrange for Caroline to bring her sewing machine when
she visits in a few days time.

We swim the next morning and then pack a picnic
lunch to take to Mulhaven. Tim announces that he plans
to spend the afternoon fishing instead. He doesn't want
to see Grandma again. He finds it too upsetting. I respond
rather sharply. 'It's not about you, Tim. You're going for
Grandma's benefit. You can't avoid things just because
they make you feel bad.'

Tim gets in the car. June, a good friend of Mum's, is
at the nursing home when we arrive. She tells me that
she visited last night and a nurse she hadn't seen before
gave Pat her Dilantin capsules – all three in her mouth at
once – just as dinner was served. It took an hour and a half
to get Pat to finish chewing and swallowing the plastic-
coated capsules, and then her meal had to be reheated
before June could feed it to her.

I show Robin and Linden the piano and receive permission to use it from the friendly lady in the Social Cen-

tre. But the staff are busy, and Mum has begun to look sleepy by the time someone finally comes to transfer her from the bed to her big Regency recliner. I wheel her to the other building and she opens her eyes briefly as the boys play their memorised pieces, but I am not sure that she understands what is going on.

On the last day of our visit, the tea lady comes by with her trolley and serves us hot beverages and cakes but leaves only a cup of orange cordial for Mum. When I question this, she consults her list and informs me that Mary is only down for a cold drink and all her food has to be mashed. I feel sorry that one of the few pleasures left to my mother has been eroded so severely. I know she can still eat normal food if the person feeding her is patient. And I feel angry about the 'Mary'. How many times do we have to tell them that despite what is written on their official forms, she has always been called Pat?

Mum's GP at Mulhaven, Dr Edwards, contacts me twice at the end of October. The first time he tells me that Pat is eating very little, her elevated cancer markers and mounting level of pain suggest that the cancer is now active throughout her body, and he thinks she has weeks rather than months to live.

My predominant response is relief. The vegetative limbo that my mother has been in since May seems to be shifting into the final phase that will release her. I send

Michael and Kathy an email relating what the doctor has told me.

I get a phone call from Michael. 'I wish you'd ring me about this kind of stuff,' he says. I apologise. He's often difficult to catch on the telephone and it hadn't occurred to me that he might find the news shocking. I had assumed we were all expecting it.

My message distresses Kathy, too. 'I went to see Pat this afternoon but I don't think my visit did her any good at all,' she tells me. 'I was feeling very upset and when I started crying she went from looking settled to looking very sad.' I try suggesting that acknowledging sad feelings is appropriate at this point, but she reiterates that her visit did her sister 'no good' and adds that going every weekend on her own is very hard. Kathy's husband and son have been refusing to accompany her, citing the stock excuses. *I can't bear to see her like that. I want to remember her how she was.*

Two days later, I receive another phone call from Dr Edwards. This time he says that Pat is getting worse faster than he'd expected, her pulse is weak, he is unable to rouse her to talk to him, and he thinks she might die within a few days.

NOVEMBER

Family and friends converge on Mulhaven. When I get

there, I am surprised to discover that my mother doesn't look much different from when I saw her three weeks earlier. She is reasonably alert and even smiles when Michael and I read her funny excerpts from *Prickle Farm*. Deb, an efficient, kind-hearted blonde who is one of our favourite nurses, intimates that the 'low' Pat had experienced over the weekend might have been due to inadequate pain relief.

Over lunch at Kathy's house, someone suggests that as we are all gathered here, we should take this opportunity to have an early birthday party for Pat, even though she will not turn sixty-six for another ten days. Kathy and Caroline immediately seize upon this as a way of protecting their sister from the realisation that our purpose in coming was to attend her death-bed.

'We'll tell her tomorrow is her birthday!'

I veto this pretence. I feel we have colluded in my mother's refusal to accept the inevitable for long enough. Everyone is suppressing their true feelings, acting as though nothing is wrong. And I think all this falsity is creating emotional distance at a time when we should be drawing as close to her as possible.

I ring Mulhaven and tell Deb about our plans for the birthday party, hoping to ensure that someone will get Mum washed and out of bed beforehand. When we arrive with the Black Forest Torte, disposable cups and plates, milk, teabags and instant coffee, we are surprised and delighted to find that a tea trolley has been ordered and a large quiet space has been prepared for us, fully set up with chairs, a bubbling urn and a table full of crockery.

But our feast has a spectre. Mum is zonked out on morphine, her face is tight and drawn, and her eyes stare uncomprehendingly. She is struggling to stay awake. I feel teary just looking at her.

Kathy lights a singing candle and it delivers a high-pitched rendition of Happy Birthday. We try to sing along but it is faster than we are. We take photos of Mum that I already know will turn out to be so ghastly that none of us will ever be able to look at them. Standing in the line to get myself a cup of coffee, I rest my head on Kathy's shoulder and say to her, 'Tell me this isn't a wake with the person still here?'

She looks utterly horrified. I realise that I should have kept the thought to myself.

I ask Deb if we can see Dr Edwards. I want to know if he has changed his mind about Mum's prognosis, so that I can decide whether to stay or go. Deb arranges for the doctor to come and speak to the family, even though it is his day off. He sits down with us and talks about the likelihood of pneumonia setting in soon, and the need to keep pain under control by steadily increasing the strength of the fentanyl patches. He thinks that Pat may still have a week or two left as her pulse has returned to normal.

Everyone tells me not to feel guilty if I decide to go home tomorrow. Genevieve is fretting for me and I have a stack of unmarked assignments sitting on my desk. I don't want to stay here for weeks, watching the clock, waiting for it to be over. I would rather go away and come back when it really is nearer the end.

Michael has already announced that he is not going to stay. I know that he is desperate to get home and placate his wife. My sister-in-law Lydia is a smart, successful woman – which is why I am always surprised when she acts like someone who is rabidly insecure. Yesterday Michael forgot to ring and wish the children goodnight; this morning he got a text message saying: 'Don't bother to call us. Other people are obviously more important than we are.' Since then she has been refusing to answer the phone. The fact that Michael has told me about this is a measure of how bewildered and upset he is. Until now, his loyalty and devotion have led him to rationalise and justify whatever she does, but even he cannot fathom how she could behave so badly when his mother is dying.

The Baptist pastor who attends Mulhaven, Peter Janz, has a close relationship with my mother. Peter has been sitting with us listening to what the doctor has to say. After the doctor leaves, he advises that now is the time to tell Pat anything in our hearts that remains unsaid. We decide that tomorrow morning we will speak to her, one at a time.

I rise early, pack my bags and drive to Alstonville. I want space and time to tell Mum how much I love her, and to say that even though her body is shutting down and she is going to die soon, she will always be with us, in our thoughts, in our memories and in the stories we tell of her. I do manage to get it all out, but Mulhaven at eight in the morning is a noisy place and I keep being interrupted by bustling nurses and clanking cleaners. Then Peter Janz arrives and whisks me off to an alcove to suggest that I encourage my father to give Pat a hug and tell her that he loves her, because blokes don't do that often enough. He keeps me there for longer than I want to be away, and by the time I get back to Mum's room, Michael and Dad are there.

Michael sends us off so he can talk to Mum alone. He tells me later that he spoke about how much he appreciated the family life she had created for us and the holidays she had worked so hard to provide. He also told her that he regretted seeing less of her over the last ten years, but he'd been busy establishing his own family.

Then Dad has his turn. He's not convinced that Mum is taking much in because she is only semiconscious. I say she probably can hear us, even if she can't respond. Last night he admitted to having some 'regrets' but didn't elaborate, apart from telling me that he and Mum discussed them a while ago and said sorry to each other.

I go in again to say goodbye before driving home. It

is hard to do. I have just told her she is dying; now I am telling her that I am leaving. I promise that I will be back next weekend.

I have been in Armidale for only three days when Kathy rings to say Pat is worse; she is almost comatose and her breathing is congested and irregular. I ask if she looks pale and if her hands and feet are cold. I have been obsessively reading up on the signs and symptoms of each stage of the dying process. I don't know why, but I have become fixated on finely calculating my departure from home so that I will arrive in time, but not too early. When Kathy reports that Pat's colour and temperature are normal, I say that maybe I don't need to come just yet. But after hanging up, I stand by the phone, irresolute. I ring Mulhaven and speak to the nurse on duty. She basically repeats what Kathy has said and then adds that my gut feeling will tell me what to do.

An hour later, I am on my way. As I approach the point where mobile phone coverage blacks out for the long stretch between Armidale and Grafton, I think to turn my mobile on and check for missed calls. Caroline has rung. She has not left a message but I can hear her saying, 'She didn't answer it,' in a sad sort of voice. This freaks me out so much that I sit by the side of the road calling first her and then Kathy, until finally one of them answers and reassures me that nothing has changed. They'd spoken to

Tim and he'd said I was coming. They just wanted to tell me to drive safely.

By eight o'clock that evening, I am standing beside my mother's bed at Mulhaven. She has her eyes half open and is breathing in an irregular sort of way, with long pauses. Caroline and Kathy return from having dinner. A woman I haven't seen for decades is with them. Judy, an old friend of Mum's from Box Hill, who became a friend of Caroline's as well when the three of them teamed up to travel around Europe in 1991. Seeing Judy here reminds me of my mother's impressive ability to keep her friendships alive even when distance and time intervene to make it difficult.

We all sit in the darkened room and talk quietly for an hour. Mum's hands and feet feel normal. I decide it probably isn't necessary to sleep in a chair beside her bed after all, and drive on to Dad's place.

Several times during the night I wake and wonder how my mother is faring. I ring Mulhaven at dawn and Jenny, the registered nurse who has been on duty since eleven o'clock tells me that Pat had a restful night. 'She's awake and alert now,' says Jenny. 'I don't know if anyone was planning to come in, but she seems to be looking for company and we're all rushing around here ... '

We'd been told yesterday that they were short-staffed. In the trailing tones of Jenny's voice, I hear sorrow that she has no time to spare for a person who may be having their last few lucid moments in this world.

Mum turns her face towards me as I walk in and seems to register my presence. She is lying on her back, breathing normally and quietly, looking peaceful. But I am not peaceful. I am up and down, checking the visitors' book; freshening up a vase by extracting the dead flowers, then having to clear up the resulting mess of fallen petals on the floor; putting on some music – 'Bach for Breakfast' – all the time aware of my shoes emitting squeaks of complaint about my restlessness.

One of the care assistants, a very large young woman called Rose, comes in and greets Pat tenderly, stroking her hair and calling her sweetheart. 'Are you going to get up and do my work so I can lie in bed for a while?' she wants to know. A slight brightening of Mum's face indicates that she has heard.

I will myself to be calmer. I sit and read *Prickle Farm* while my mother drifts in and out of consciousness. A few times I look up and catch her in one of her awake moments and I smile and speak to her.

As the day goes on, Dad, Caroline, Judy and Heather come in and take turns spending time in the room. Michael rings at sunset for the latest news and lists all the reasons why he is not intending to come down. He is overseeing the finishing touches on their new house and needs to be on site to coordinate the activities of the various contractors. Lydia is doing an important presentation at work in a few days time and will need him to look after the children. Besides, he has said his goodbyes to Mum already.

The next morning, Dr Edwards tells us that Pat has contracted pneumonia. 'I'm going to let it run its course,' he says.

'How long will that take?' I ask.

'Could be thirty-six hours. Could be a week.'

This seems like a very broad range to me. I understand why he has decided not to delay the inevitable with antibiotics, but I am concerned about the fact that Mum is now wide awake and on her third day of having nothing to eat or drink. We are not supposed to give her water because she can no longer swallow, but she is obviously thirsty. When we swab her mouth to ease the dryness, she clamps her jaws around the moist little green stick and sucks ferociously.

'Could she die of dehydration in that time? Should she be on a drip?'

'No,' says the doctor. 'It will be the pneumonia that kills her. And it would be cruel to put her on a drip at this point.'

I am starting to wonder what has become of Dad, when he arrives bearing an armful of freshly blooming pink roses from Mum's garden. These flowers are special, a legacy of beauty from my mother's childhood. The plant was originally a cutting from a climbing rose treasured by my grandmother. I am touched that Dad has thought to bring them.

Deb confides that she had been shocked by my mother's reaction to the news that she had pneumonia and would not receive treatment for it. She had expected that Mum would have come to terms with her impending death by now.

'She doesn't change her mind easily,' I say. 'She's stubborn.'

I ring Michael to tell him about the pneumonia and to marvel at the fact that Mum's fighting spirit is still rejecting the idea of dying even as her body is shutting down its last remaining functions. 'I don't think she's ever going to accept it,' I say.

'Well, I wouldn't either.'

His comment makes me wonder why I am clinging to the expectation that Mum should meet this coming death with serenity. Why can't she *rage, rage against the dying of the light* if she wants to?

I walk back into her room. No one else is there. I rest my elbows on the rails of the bed and catch her eye. 'It looks like you're going down fighting,' I say. 'Deb was surprised to find out that you're not accepting what's happening but I explained that you've always been bloody-minded.'

Her face quirks into a smile.

That evening, I return to an empty house and sit aimlessly, feeling bereft. Dad comes home soon afterwards but he is clearly overwrought and his presence makes me feel worse. Walking in the door, he shrieks at Monty, their aged, over-weight Labrador, who is trying to come inside in search of his dinner. A few moments later, I hear him yelling through the window at the visiting bull, because it is monopolising the food laid out for the cows. A desperate desire to escape rises like acid in my throat but I assume self-effacing camouflage and we pass a normal evening together, except for me crying over photos of Mum while Dad is having his shower. When Kathy rings, I tell her all about it and she suggests that I should have given my father a cuddle instead of trying to blend into the furniture.

'But when he carries on like this, it makes me feel four years old again,' I whine, looking for sympathy, invoking shared memories of a childhood agitated by my father's angry hysterics.

'Perhaps you could try to get past that,' she says. Although I don't find this comment particularly useful at the time, the idea stays with me.

As Dad and I walk towards Mum's room the following morning we meet a nurse who tells us that Pat's condition dipped quite low during the night, but she is very alert now. However, when we take up our positions on either side of the bed, Mum gives no indication of noticing that we are there. It takes me a minute to realise that she is listening intently to the CD that is playing – 'Hymns of Praise.' Then I think I hear her say something.

'What was that?' I ask my father.

'She's singing,' he says.

I turn to Mum for confirmation. 'Are you singing?'

'Yes,' she responds.

I am overjoyed to hear her voice again. Dad seems not to appreciate how special this singing and speaking is; he continues to talk over the top of her. I turn up the volume on the CD player, wishing I could turn him down. I go out to the notice board to see if there is a church service today and am thrilled to find that there is a Baptist one on at ten o'clock. I arrange for Mum to be transferred to a chair so she can attend.

I ring Caroline and announce that Mum is talking today. She is as excited and incredulous as I am. She says she'll be there soon and will bring Kathy.

During the church service, Dad sits next to Mum and they share a hymn book. I am surprised to hear Dad singing 'What a friend we have in Jesus' with great gusto. He says he remembers it from Sunday School. Mum doesn't sing. It looks like she is in pain. Later we will learn that she has broken a rib, possibly when the care assistants were getting her out of bed.

Back in her room after the service, I observe that one of

the cleaners manages to elicit a soft 'Fine' from Mum when he asks in an exuberant voice how she is today. The loud friendliness of some of the staff, and their determination to get a smile out of Pat even though she is dying, make me feel uncomfortable. I am wondering whether enforced jollity is a form of bullying when the plump girl, Rose, comes bustling in. She seems to have only one joke, and that afternoon she runs it past us again.

'Pat, are you going to get up and do all my work so I can lie down there for a while?'

I mention that I'd heard her make that offer before. I hope she hasn't been saying it to Mum every day for the past three months.

That night, I try to persuade Michael to come and see Mum again. 'What if she asks for you, at the end? What do we tell her? "Michael's not here because his new floor coverings are more important?"'

I regret that crack as soon as the words leave my mouth, but I hate the thought of Mum yearning for her son and dying disappointed. And after I hang up, another disturbing thought strikes me. It is entirely possible that she has forgotten every loving word Michael said during his last visit.

Once again I make my early morning phone call to Mulhaven, half dreading, half longing to hear that my mother's condition has changed. But no – she passed a restful night and is awake and alert.

Michael calls half an hour later and I set my breakfast aside to marshal my new argument. 'Yes, you've said your goodbyes and told her everything you need to. But you know what her memory is like. What if she doesn't remember what you said? Or doesn't even remember that you were here at all?'

He says he'll have to talk to Lydia. He rings back and tells me he has booked a seat on the bus.

Dad and I arrive at Mulhaven to find Mum's door is closed. Deb is in there, conferring with the care assistants who have been doing a bed-bath. They let us in and show us a protuberance at the bottom of Pat's ribcage. Deb explains that the bones around the sternum may be chalky from the tumours and the rib might have just popped, perhaps while Pat was coughing, perhaps when she was moved yesterday.

Deb leaves to ring the doctor. Mum tries to talk to us. We sit on the edge of our chairs, hanging on every sound coming from that poor parched mouth, but we cannot make out what she is trying to say. Her tongue is thick and coated with sticky white mucus. I swab it with the sponge on a stick. It is impregnated with bicarbonate of soda and makes the water turn cloudy. I wish I could give her cool, clear water for a proper drink.

Kathy, Caroline and Judy arrive. Mum keeps trying to

talk, we keep straining to understand. It is desperately sad. She is holding the lump on her midriff with her hand, occasionally grimacing with spasms of pain.

Deb comes back. The doctor is not going to come. He said they should use pain relief to manage the broken rib, because strapping it might make another one pop on the other side. Deb tells Mum that she is going to give her an injection of morphine, and goes away to fetch it.

Very clearly, Mum says, 'I don't want that stuff. I want to stay awake.'

Three of us form a deputation to head off the morphine. Deb agrees, reluctantly. She administers Rivotril instead, saying it might have a relaxing effect. Mum keeps looking around. She says something about Michael.

Caroline rings Michael and leaves a message on his phone. Can he drive down instead of catching the bus? His mother is asking for him and refusing pain relief because she wants to stay alert until he comes. He sends back a text message to say that he is leaving immediately.

Mum holds out against the morphine and is awake when Michael arrives. Her whole face lightens when he enters the room. A couple of hours later she has the injection and we leave her to sleep.

The next day, Mum slips into a comatose state with her eyes rolled back and her breathing shallow and irregular. Caroline, Kathy, Michael and I decide that the end is near and that we will stay overnight at Mulhaven. We pass long hours listening to the fierce, dry intakes of breath in the darkened room. Mum is so desiccated from a week without water that even her death rattle has evaporated. I am plagued by windy pains in the stomach but manage to doze in various places – on the floor wrapped in a quilt, sitting in the recliner, and briefly on a sofa bed that we discover in one of the lounge rooms. At midnight Mum clocks up another year of age. It is the 11th of November, her birthday. She is sixty-six. Three of the care assistants have stayed back an hour after the end of their shift in order to celebrate this moment. They have to be at work again by seven a.m. so this is sweet of them.

We schedule breaks for each other during the day but although I return to Dad's place and lie down on my bed, I don't manage to sleep. On the second night of the vigil, I spend the hours from one until four awake while Michael slumbers on the floor and Caroline and Kathy sleep in the lounge room. I move from one uncomfortable chair to another, listening to Olivia Newton-John singing about being stronger than before, standing up to relieve my stiffness and swaying with tiredness, feeling that I can't go on doing this for much longer.

I am engulfed by misery as I watch my mother, so wasted and broken, such a tiny bony bundle but still shaking the bed with her desperate, pointless breaths. I lean close and whisper, 'You can stop. We love you but it's time to let go.'

A nurse comes with another shot of morphine and as she walks into the room her phone rings loudly. Immediately, Mum's eyes fly open and her body spasms in a seizure that lasts for several minutes. I see that she is conscious and terrified. The nurse struggles to put drops under her tongue as she bucks.

I walk down to the lounge room and wake Kathy. She puts her arms around me as I confess how hard I am finding it all. 'I hate the fact that I'm sitting there wishing she'd stop breathing,' I gasp tearfully.

Kathy goes stiff. 'What do you wish?' she asks coldly.

She tells me that she doesn't wish Pat would stop breathing. She sits there still praying for the miracle. She is glad that Pat is peaceful. She is happy to let her do things in her own time.

I feel crushed and contemptible. Fancy wishing my own mother dead! I get into the bed that Kathy has vacated, tears continuing to roll down my face. I start to think about leaving – picking up my stuff and walking out to the car and not coming back – but I tell myself this would be indefensible.

Caroline clambers out of the recliner and comes over to me.

'Can you understand why I want this to be over?'

'Yes, sweetheart.'

'Kathy doesn't. She's angry at me.'

Caroline makes soothing noises. She says everyone is

struggling to cope with what is happening. Then she becomes theological. She can't understand how suffering like my mother's can be reconciled with the idea of the Christian god. Eventually she leaves me to sleep. I manage two lots of half an hour before packing up the bed at six thirty a.m.

I consider going straight back to Dad's to eat and sleep but Michael has started talking about going home on the bus today so we need to organise the telephone lists. We have decided to divvy up the job of notifying the hundred or so people who will want to be informed about Pat's death, when it happens. We are busy sorting through the names when Mum has another seizure. Once again, I am stricken to see that she is fully with us, wide awake and frightened as the seizure shakes her. When it finally ends, her expression is fixed and she doesn't breathe for an age.

The care assistant who came running when we pressed the bell strokes Mum's face during the not-breathing phase and murmurs, 'Mary, come on Mary.'

I can hardly bear it, the tenderness and the wrong name together.

'Oh, please don't call her that!' I moan.

All day there are bells and running feet heading for my mother's room. I appeal to Michael not to leave. I say we've seen how the seizures pull Mum out of her peaceful unconscious state and into terror and pain. Someone does need to be with her all the time, or she could be going through them alone, without anyone realising. I tell him that I am already frazzled from lack of sleep and don't know if I can do another night duty. If he leaves, it is more load that the rest of us will have to carry, and it is hard enough already. He says that he'll talk to Lydia.

I decide to go for a swim. Chris rings me as I am walking to the pool. I tell him that Mum seems weaker, her breathing not so forceful as before, but still like the Duracell bunny, she keeps on keeping on. He suggests that it might be kinder to put a pillow over her face, but I vehemently reject that idea. Apart from knowing that I would never be able to do it, I am well aware my mother's most ardent desire is to live, not die.

Michael agrees to stay another night. I go to Dad's place and sleep a blessed eight hours and return to Mulhaven the next morning. Kathy has great dark shadows under her eyes; she jokes that it is a new way of applying makeup. Dad and I send the others away to rest, and we manage most of the day shift together even though Dad admits he doesn't like being there, sitting and watching while Mum is dying. He says it makes him feel like a ghoul. I tell him that Mum would not want to die alone and that we all appreciate his perseverance.

'I'm proud that you're willing to help us do this,' I say. 'You know, once I wouldn't have believed you were capable of it.'

'I guess I'm mellowing with age,' he replies.

Perhaps he is. Certainly, I will continue to be amazed by the changes in him in the months and years ahead. After Mum's death, he will surprise us all with the intensity of his grief. He will assuage his loneliness by reaching out to people with acts of kindness and consideration; he will curb his irritability and improve his relationships; he will become someone who remembers birthdays, someone who gives his time to community service organisations. After Mum's death, he will become someone who is much easier to love.

I notice that Mum's seizures seem to be happening just before her morphine is due. She is also crying out with pain whenever she is moved. I ask for the pain relief to be increased and am told that the doctor will need to authorise it. Later, we learn that her fentanyl patches were not changed at their usual time because the pharmacy had run out of stock. Only the morphine injections were working and they were supposed to be a top-up. One side effect of the pain is that it seems to bring Mum closer to consciousness. From the little flickers on her face, we get the impression that she is listening to us talk.

Deb comes back on duty on Tuesday. When she'd left on Friday, she hadn't expected to see Mum again. When she walks into the room, Mum sets up an almighty groaning noise. We are all amazed. I suggest that Mum is trying to communicate with Deb, to let her know that she is hurting and trusts her to do something about it. The nurses yesterday had fobbed me off, saying that pain at this stage was unavoidable. Deb rings Dr Edwards but he says he is not coming in and can't authorise the extra morphine electronically as their computer systems are down. So Deb marches up the hill to his surgery and stands there until he signs the forms.

The long vigil ends as day fades into evening. Caroline and I have just finished eating our dinner, a fragrant mix of meat and vegetables that Heather has brought in for us. Mum is lying on the bed, flat on her back, her mouth open, deeply unconscious. Over the course of the afternoon, her hands and feet have developed the purple blotches that we have been anticipating for so long.

Caroline and I sit with our empty plates on our laps and chat easily. We swap stories about encounters with snakes. We laugh and reminisce and for a few moments we forget what we are doing here. Then Caroline notices it is seven o'clock, free-talk time on her mobile, and goes outside to phone her daughters.

Left alone with Mum, I feel guilty about how we have been ignoring her. I stand up and stroke her hair. I speak to her, assuming she can still hear. I say I'm sorry, that we had just been distracting ourselves from the sadness of the situation.

I have read that dying people can feel disorientated, so

I mention that it is the 14th of November, 2006 and that she turned sixty-six a few days ago. I tell her again what a wonderful mother she was, and remind her that Michael was here earlier and he'd told her how much he appreciated the family life she had created and the holidays she had taken us on.

Mum's arms and legs feel cold so I fetch a soft blanket and snuggle it around her. I watch her taking tiny sips of air for a few moments and then say, 'What little breaths, sweetheart. And how blue your fingers are.'

I cry. I give her a kiss. I say I love her and I will always miss her.

There is a gentle knock at the door. It is one of Mum's church friends, Christine. I ask her to sit with Mum while I go to my car to fetch more tissues. As I am leaving, Christine says, 'Did you see that? I was just stroking her cheek and she closed her mouth.'

When I come back to the room a few minutes later, Christine says softly, 'I don't think Pat's breathing.'

We watch until I know she is not going to take another breath. She has died, very peacefully, with my words in her ears and Christine's fingers on her face.

Some names have been changed in this story

Further reading

In the course of writing 'A Hospital Bed at Home', I discovered many books and internet-based resources that I wish I had known about when I first became a caregiver. This list contains those that I found most enlightening, moving and informative.

Personal stories

Addison, S 2001, *Mother Lode: Stories of home life and home death*, University of Queensland Press, St Lucia, Queensland. *Passionately and poetically written, this memoir tells the life and death of Susan Addison's teenage son.*

Brennan, F 2007, 'A doctor's notebook', *Griffith Review*, Edition 17 – Staying Alive, at http://www.griffithreview.com/edition17/78-memoir/124-brennan17.html *A collection of Dr Frank Brennan's moving tales of his work as a palliative care specialist.*

Garner, H 2008, *The Spare Room*, Text Publishing.
In this novel heavily based on her own experiences, Garner provides a searingly honest portrait of a caregiver's thoughts and reactions.

Hender, M 2004, *Saying Goodbye – Stories of caring for the dying*, ABC Books, Sydney.
Portrays the experiences of ten caregivers with a focus on the positive and spiritual aspects of the situation.

Lloyd, V 2008, *The Young Widow's Book of Home Improvement: A true story of love and renovation*, University of Queensland Press, St Lucia, Qld.
About love, loss and grief – and putting your house in order.

Palliative Care Australia 2005, *A Journey Lived: A collection of personal stories from carers*, PCA, at http://www.palliativecare.org.au/Portals/46/resources/AJourneyLived.pdf
Eight brief accounts of supporting a loved one towards death with the help of palliative care services.

Rieff, D 2008, *Swimming in a Sea of Death: A son's memoir*, Simon & Schuster, New York.
David Rieff, the son of Susan Sontag, says he felt impelled to be his mother's chief cheerleader as she forced herself through a series of gruelling, futile treatments in order to avoid dying.

Rose, P 2001, *Rose Boys*, Allen & Unwin, Sydney.
An award-winning family memoir about suffering, devotion, dependence and mortality.

Valenta, T 2007, *Remember me Mrs V? Caring for my Wife: Her Alzheimer's and others' stories*, Michelle Anderson Publishing, Melbourne.
Former journalist Tom Valenta describes his own and others' experiences of caring for a loved one with Alzheimer's disease.

Wyndham, S 2008, *Life in his Hands: The true story of a neurosurgeon and a pianist*, Pan Macmillan, Sydney.
The true story of controversial neurosurgeon Dr Charlie Teo and one of his most high-profile and tragic cases, young pianist Aaron McMillan.

Informative

Advance Care Directive Association Inc 2013, *My Health, My Future, My Choice: An Advance Care Directive for New South Wales*, at http://www.advancecaredirectives.org.au
Combines a workbook with the form, and explains the issues and terms in a way that a layperson can understand.

Anastasios, Andrew 2007, *Dying to Know: Bringing death to life*, Pilotlight Australia, Prahan, Victoria.

A delightful, thought-provoking little book of illustrations, epigrams and wisdom.

Barbato, M 2002, *Caring for the Dying*, McGraw-Hill Sydney.
Written by a doctor with forty years of experience in palliative care, this handbook is a fount of clear, useful information and an insightful guide to the emotional aspects of caring for people as they are dying.

Barnard, D, Towers, A, Boston, P & Lambrinidou, Y 2000, *Crossing Over: Narratives of palliative care*, Oxford University Press Inc, New York.
Richly detailed case studies of particular patients and their families, written by palliative care researchers.

Carers Australia 2007, *Carer's Handbook: A practical Australian guide to caring for people who are sick, elderly or have a disability*, Dorling Kindersley Australasia, Camberwell, Vic.
Published in conjunction with St John's Ambulance Service, a fully illustrated guide with comprehensive advice on all aspects of home-based caring.

Four Corners – *A Good Death* program web site:
http://www.abc.net.au/4corners/content/2010/s2810506.htm
Contains the video and transcript of this excellent ABC TV docu-

mentary about palliative care, as well as many links to further information.

Marriott, H 2006, *The Selfish Pig's Guide to Caring*, Time Warner Books, London.
A humorous, irreverent look at some of the taboo subjects of caregiving, including resentment, sexual frustration, incontinence and the occasional desire to push your loved one down the stairs, written by a man whose wife deteriorated over many years from Huntington's disease.

Palliative Care Australia web site:
http://www.palliativecare.org.au
The peak national organisation working to foster and promote the delivery of quality care at the end of life.

Palliative Care Australia 2004, 'The hardest thing we have ever done': Full report of the national inquiry into the social impact of caring for terminally ill people, PCA, Canberra, at
http://www.palliativecare.org.au/Portals/46/
The%20hardest%20thing.pdf
The first section highlights the challenges and difficulties faced by family carers; the second section analyses public submissions from individual carers, service providers and support organisations.

Wakely, M 2008, *Sweet Sorrow: A beginner's guide to death*, Melbourne University Press, Carlton, Victoria.
Mark Wakely embarks on a personal crusade to explore the issues, practices and customs surrounding the end of life.

World Health Organization 2007, *WHO definition of palliative care*, at http://www.who.int/cancer/palliative/definition/en/
The World Health Organisation's definition of palliative care.

Zuger, A 2008, 'A fight for life consumes both mother and son', *The New York Times*, January 29, at http://www.nytimes.com/2008/01/29/health/29book.html
A penetrating review of David Rieff's memoir by a medical doctor who says Susan Sontag set a new benchmark for 'a bad death'.

ACKNOWLEDGEMENTS

This book was written as part of a PhD in creative writing, and so I owe an enormous debt to my knowledgeable, helpful and enthusiastic supervisors, Professor Donna Lee Brien from CQUniversity and Dr Glenda Parmenter from the University of New England. Thanks also to the postgraduate comrades who provided support and acted as sounding boards, especially Helena Pastor, Peter Mitchell, Siobhan McHugh, Sandra Lindemann, Helen Gildfind, John Gintowt, Susan Currie, Sam Carroll, Rachel Franks and Sandra Arnold. Thank you also to Dr Nicole Gerrand, Wendy Mulligan, Sue Adams, Derene Anderson, Lynne O'Brien and Marilyn McCarthy from the Hunter New England Health service.

For their insightful, constructive feedback on my work, I would also like to express my gratitude to Professor Jen Webb, Dr Frank Brennan, Petrea King, Barbara Burton, Merle Goldsmith and Jan Wyles. Warm thanks to my graphic designer friend, Trish Donald, who did a beautiful job of the cover, and my son Robin Hutchinson and mother-in-law Liz Hutchinson for their careful proofreading. And love and kisses to the rest of my family, especially my sweetly supportive husband, Chris.

Finally, and most importantly, I acknowledge the fascinating, thoughtful, inspiring people who agreed to share their lives with me. Their generosity and patience are the foundation upon which this book rests. Thank you for working so hard to help me turn your precious memories into these narrative non-fiction stories.

www.ingramcontent.com/pod-product-compliance
Lightning Source LLC
Chambersburg PA
CBHW051416090426
42737CB00014B/2698